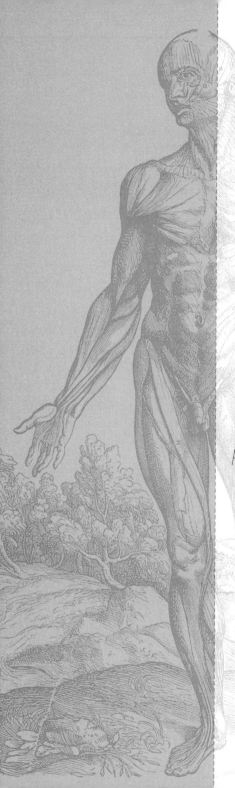

FIRST CUT

A SEASON
IN THE HUMAN
ANATOMY LAB

D0370091

ALBERT HOWARD CARTER III

PICADOR USA
NEW YORK

Picador® USA is a registered trademark and is used by St. Martin's Press under license from Pan Books Limited.

For information on Picador USA Reading Group Guides, as well as ordering, please contact the Trade Marketing department at St. Martin's Press.
Phone: 1-800-221-7945 extension 488
Fax: 212-677-7456
E-mail: trademarketing@stmartins.com

Frontispiece engraving, "The Third Plate of the Muscles," from J. B. deC. M. Saunders and Charles D. O'Malley, *The Illustrations from the Works of Andreas Vesalius of Brussels* (New York: Dover Publications, Inc.), page 97. Edition published in 1973 by arrangement with The World Publishing Company.

Design by Maureen Troy

Library of Congress Cataloging-in-Publication Data

Carter, Albert Howard.
   First cut : a season in the human anatomy lab / Albert Howard Carter, III.
      p. cm.
   ISBN 0-312-19546-x
   1. Human dissection—Georgia—Atlanta. 2. Human ana-
tomy—Study and teaching (Graduate)—Georgia—Atlanta. 3.
Emory University. School of Medicine. 1. Title.
QM33.5.C37 1997
611'.0071—dc21   97-20909
                                              CIP

First Picador USA Paperback Edition: September 1998

10 9 8 7 6 5 4 3 2 1

"Carter's depiction of the human anatomy course will arouse nostalgia in any health-care professional who has endured this traditional rite of passage. For the uninitiated, *First Cut* provides a glimpse into an otherwise closed world of exploration and discovery."

—*Humane Health Care International*

"A warmly engaging, cheerful and utterly winning book...as engrossing as any novel, as thoughtful as the most searching memoir, as suggestive as any contemporary scientific essay."

—Fred Chappell, *The Raleigh News & Observer*

"The reactions of Carter and the students make interesting reading. Their personalities come through in their individual and collective actions and utterances."

—*The Roanoke Times*

"Carter provides insight into a critical aspect of medical training, and an unusually intimate, even arresting, view of the bodies we have and the bodies we will become."

—*Publishers Weekly*

"With humor, compassion and wisdom, *First Cut* offers thoughts on what it means to be a doctor."

—*St. Petersburg Times*

"Clear depiction of what medical students must do to learn anatomy."

—*Kirkus Reviews*

"This glimpse into a world foreign to most...is fascinating."

—*Columbus Dispatch*

"Daring, detailed and humanistic...With a clear and unjaded eye, Carter not only captures the macabre atmosphere, but also the body's majesty."

—*The Tampa Tribune*

This book is dedicated to:

*Persons who have contributed a human body for medical
education or research; also their families;*

*Persons who dedicate time and effort to learn human anatomy,
first-year medical students in particular; and*

*Teachers of anatomy, who faithfully lecture, tutor,
and encourage students year after year.*

CONTENTS

PART I
COMMENCING TO CUT

PART II
INTO INTIMACIES

PART III
FROM CADAVER TO CARCASS TO
REINCORPORATION

LIST OF FIGURES

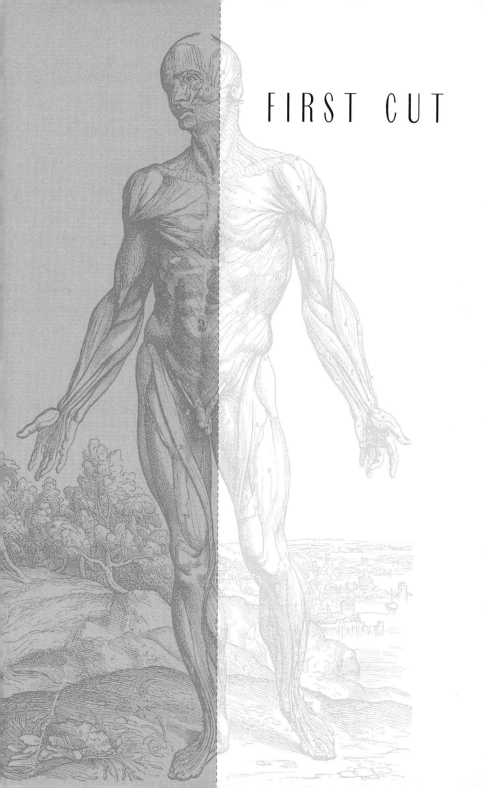

FIRST CUT

INTRODUCTION

· · ·

THE HUMAN ANATOMY lab at a medical school is usually unmarked. Its doors are typically solid wood; if there is a window in the door, it is made of frosted glass. The anatomy lab is a world apart, a place held separate by custom, ethics, and even taboo. Such separation is due to various reasons: confidentiality and propriety, as well as historical influences from some seven hundred years ago, when the Catholic Church said that bodies should not be dismembered after death. At a deeper level, our attitudes toward the dead are colored by our universal fears of illness and death itself. Popular images of Dr. Frankenstein, madly cutting and sewing body parts together, reflect some of these fears. How are first-year medical students to understand their transition through this door, from the normal world to the world of cutting up dead people? We live in a culture that has ambiguous attitudes about the body: on the one hand, we idealize it; on the other, we are afraid of it.

When I was a kid—and even throughout my teens—I wanted to be a doctor. In America this profession had high status: economic power, social recognition, and something more, an intimacy with other persons, both psychological and physical. I was briefly pre-med in college; I got through chemistry and calculus with only moderate success, and I saw fellow students who had a motivation that I did not. Since I had also wanted to be a teacher and loved reading, the world of words easily seduced me. I graduated in humanities and went on for graduate work in English and comparative literature. Still, even as I approached middle age, I had the nagging sense that I might have become a physician. There are, in fact, programs for converting Ph.D.s into M.D.s, and I have fantasized about that possibility for myself. Part of me headed for the anatomy lab to see whether I should have—or perhaps still could—become a doctor.

If you live long enough, however, sometimes you can still travel roads not taken, often in surprising ways. In the early eighties I was at the Center for Bioethics at the Kennedy Institute of Ethics of Georgetown University, where I learned that literature and medicine was an emerging field. One of the reasons I had specialized in literature was a search for intimacy with others, whether characters, authors, or fellow readers who were willing to share what they observed in texts. Through poems, plays, stories, novels, and even nonfiction, I could see what was important to other persons, what they desired and feared, and how they suffered, fell in love, cherished their dreams, survived tragedy, and faced death. Many of these intense states stem from physical illness or personal injury; indeed, literature is full of symbolism of illness, from the misery of Job to the plague of Oedipus Rex, from the dwarfism of Grass's Oskar to the illness and death of Tolstoy's Ivan Ilych. To be ill is to lose the ordering structures of life, to lose energy and a sense of the possible, while gaining understanding of pain and despair. Physicians who were also writers had a double perspective on the intimacies of bodies and minds; I investigated Rabelais, Chekhov, A. Conan Doyle, Céline, Bulgakov, William Carlos Williams, Walker Percy, Richard Selzer, and John Stone. Both Keats and Gertrude Stein studied medicine. What did they know, from their training and experience, that other writers wouldn't know? What was there about the physicality of human flesh, in its strength and weakness, that illuminated the human condition?

As I pursued the "medical humanities," as this new field was called, I observed an autopsy, a liver transplant, and other surgeries, as well as various hospital treatments and clinical visits. I took courses in emergency medicine and became a state-certified Emergency Medical Technician; I enjoyed learning the terminology, the procedures, and the professional values of this training, even though I have never actually worked as an EMT. Instead I became a pastoral care volunteer in a combination trauma center and emergency room in 1988 and have continued that calling up to this writing. I have seen there a wide variety of illnesses, accidents, and the harm humans can inflict on each other or on themselves. I have talked to hundreds of patients about their hopes and fears. I admired the technicians, nurses, and physicians who dealt with these patients, and—even in spite of my weakness in the sciences—I persisted in wondering whether I might ever join any of these professions. Helpful doctors would explain X rays and various other bits of medical information and reasoning. They impressed me with their humanity, their efficiency, and their technical skill. How did they first learn about the human body and what's inside our skin?

The purpose of this book is to take the reader into the anatomy lab and to look over the students' shoulders as they cut, discover, and slowly come to understand working with a cadaver. The particular course described here is the Human Anatomy course for first-year medical students at Emory University in Atlanta, where I was an observer for sixteen weeks during a fall semester. Watching the students work and talking with them, I collected material that became this account. Yes, there are repulsive aspects of the lab, and it is often tedious, a place of seemingly endless, exacting labor. But these qualities pale before the discoveries the students make regarding the bodies they are assigned. In brief, the lab is a place where the magnificence of the human body becomes clear, and med students learn reverence for, we might say, their first patient.

As a professor of literature, I am interested in stories, images, language, and the ways students talked about their experience. I tend to perceive the anatomy world in literary terms, and I see narrative and essay as the best ways for me to describe and interpret the complex world of the lab. I have taught bioethics, literature and medicine, and, with a biologist, "The Human Body as an Environment." For me, narrative is a way to explore unusual worlds, even worlds of extremity. I have written elsewhere about the recent development of the living will, for example, as a kind of narrative that allows us to consider our deaths. In working with Anton Chekhov's short story *Ward Six,* I have felt the dilemma of the physician who is suspended between the world of the well and the world of the sick. In Chekhov's story the physician, whose duty is to care for insane patients, goes insane himself and is committed to the grubby hospital for which he had responsibility. Modern analogues for doctors include alcoholism, substance abuse, chronic stress, depression, and even suicide—all of which happen to physicians at a higher rate than to the population at large. Thus the question, "How does a physician learn to deal with disability and death?" is not an idle aesthetic or philosophical question.

As the Emory course unrolled I became aware of more subconscious motivations that brought me to this strange world. Was I ghoulish? Voyeuristic? Upon reflection, I don't think so. Certainly there was the mechanical interest in the human body per se—what's inside? how does it look "backstage"? and what are the slings and levers I used to study in anatomical drawings? I wanted to know how this corpus, our mobile home, all fits together. I wanted to know something more of the mysteries of life and death. I also wanted to see how first-year med students went through various rites of passage, including the receiving of a human body as a gift they would dissect in order to learn.

A more general conclusion is that I (and others) like to explore the unusual, the unknown, the extreme. As I have observed in the emergency room, many medical people enjoy working at the margins, the limits of human health and experience. Physicians, nurses, and paramedics test their mettle daily, working with difficult cases that arrive by ambulance and helicopter, and I talk with patients and their families as they deal with sudden calamities. My sense of humanity grows as I participate in this world. Indeed, part of me envies medical workers—what a calling, what a chance to make a difference in someone's life.

But the strongest impetus pushing me toward the human anatomy lab only gradually became clear to me as the semester progressed. In 1970, my father, also a literature professor, was diagnosed with glioblastoma, a particularly malignant form of brain cancer. He was but fifty-six years old. As my family rallied around him during his long, slow decline, we saw his journey from health to death, the disintegration of his body and mind, the kindness of our family doctor but also the limits of his skills and, of course, the limits of all the other physicians who treated him and could not save his life. My father willed his body for medical research. Upon his death the funeral home sent his body to a medical school some 150 miles away—and that was all we knew. What happened to his body? Whom did it serve? We assumed it was used for the education of future physicians, but never had any definite notion. I wondered for many years what had happened to his body. I'm not a strong believer in the comfort of grave sites or gravestones, but I felt a yearning to know something of "where he ended up." Watching these young students begin their journey into the human body, I was searching for my lost father.

A Note on Confidentiality: Confidentiality about the cadavers has been carefully observed; I have changed details, causes of death, and more so that in no case can the remains of an actual person be identified.

—ALBERT HOWARD CARTER III
Eckerd College
St. Petersburg, Florida

PART I

COMMENCING
TO CUT

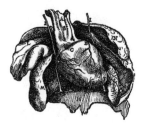

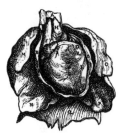

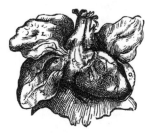

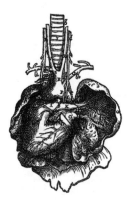

THE HEART: FOUR VIEWS

(Figure 1)

THIS WOODCUT IS from the revolutionary *De humani corporis fabrica* of Andreas Vesalius (1543), often called simply *De fabrica,* pages 565, 566. (See "A Glimpse of Vesalius" and "Cutting with Vesalius" below.)

This and other woodcuts below are taken, by permission, from *The Illustrations from the Works of Andreas Vesalius*, eds. J. B. deC. M. Saunders and Charles D. O'Malley (New York: Dover Publications, Inc., 1973), p. 181. Some of my captions owe to the commentary of these editors; future citations will be to Saunders and O'Malley.

Until William Harvey, Vesalius (and everyone else in the West) followed Galen, who believed circulation was an "ebb-and-flow" motion of the blood. In the ancient view, the heart was basically a two-chambered organ, which required blood to "sweat" through the interventricular septum.

Although Vesalius didn't solve the puzzle of circulation through the heart, his dissection shows the attached blood vessels, valves ("guardian membranes," he called them), and the "chordae tendinae," the tendinous cords that anchor the valves or, in the common (and accurate) phrase, the "heartstrings."

A HEART IN HAND

• • •

THE ANATOMY BOOKS make it sound so simple. To remove the heart, you cut through the pericardia (the two tissue layers around the heart), you make sure the eight major blood vessels are completely severed, and then you lift the heart out of the chest. For the first-year med students in the anatomy lab, however, everything becomes complicated: the fine cutting in a crowded area, the hope of a good grade, the fear of "screwing up the dissection," and the thought that this heart was beating, strongly and warmly, in a living human being some weeks or even days ago. The med students cut slowly, some taking up to two hours to remove the heart from their cadaver.

I'm in one of the lab's four rooms to watch these students dissect. In this room there are six tables bearing six embalmed bodies of people who have died in the past year. At each table there are, usually, two students of the Human Anatomy course. At Table 4, however, there is only one student, Karl Jacobs. A quick worker, he is the first to have a heart entirely removed from the body. I watch him cut the last blood vessel and pull the heart up and out. For a moment he stares at it in the palm of his hand, then suddenly raises it over his head in an exaggerated gesture of triumph. Lights flash off his glasses; his lab-coated arm is a dramatic white column. He roars out "Ha-haaaaa!"—the very image of a deranged scientist in a Hollywood thriller. Karl makes a huge grimace, as if he were a monster ready to bite right into this grayish but recognizable human heart.

Everyone else in the lab stares at this, the first heart in hand and the first truly theatrical gesture of the course. Up to today, students have been sober, timorous, in awe of this place and its strange proceedings. The five other dissecting teams envy Karl's progress and, perhaps, his unabashed outlook.

"Just like the Aztec priests!" a woman calls out appreciatively from across the room.

"Those Aztec guys must have been *good*—you know, *strong,*" another student says. "To bust through the ribs and sternum, all these tissues." He gestures at the wreckage he is simultaneously creating and ordering in his own cadaver.

"Yeah—and fast," another adds. "The victims were alive, remember. The idea was to get the heart out while it was still beating."

I shiver briefly, recalling the Diego Rivera mosaics in Mexico City that re-created such primal rites. Although I'm across the aisle at another table, my eyes keep looking at this heart, Karl, and the new cavity in the chest of the spindly dead man lying face up. Now Karl examines the heart, turning it over in his hands. He trims up around it, pats it with paper towels, and starts to identify the coronary arteries. Soon he sets it down and turns to the chest cavity. But he has seen me staring.

"Come take a look," he invites.

I walk across the aisle to look at this complex thing, meaty, but punched with holes. I lean forward in my starched lab coat, my hands clasped behind me. About the size and shape of a fist, the heart lies on a paper towel. The color of cardiac muscle is somewhere between red and brown, but there are also bands of yellow fat and eight scattered holes, through which I glimpse the four chambers that pump our blood. Under the diagonal bands of fat lie portions of the coronary arteries; I can see them circling down from the top of the heart, vaguely like the "crown" that the word *coronary* suggests. So, I think, these are the faithful fellows you don't want to clog with fat.

"Go ahead, pick it up: it even fits real well," Karl says. I place my gloved hand over the heart and grasp it gingerly. When it doesn't collapse, I gently tighten my fingers around it. *This odd thing pumps in my chest right now,* I think. I turn my hand over, and the heart settles into my palm perfectly—just as Karl said.

"Hey, you're right," I say, and he smiles, a beginner in anatomy, but already a teacher to me.

I find the weight of the heart paradoxical: as a chunk of interlocking muscle, it has some heft. As a shell of meat with four empty chambers and eight holes, it feels light.

Karl is busy in the chest cavity. I look around the room. Ten other students work intently on dissecting hearts from their cadavers. I forget the smells, the tedium, the strange sights of the anatomy lab. I am glad to be in this strange place where the veils of the human body are pushed aside so we can see the secrets within; I am glad to look over the shoulders of these young people, full of energy, faith, and commitment. This is an odd place for an English professor on leave from his college, far away from home. How did I get here? Why?

MEETING CADAVERS
· · ·

HE OPENING OF the course seemed like a series of thresholds to adventure. Late August in Atlanta is steamy hot; the sun dazzles, even on the green-forested hills of Emory University. I have come here for several reasons. Ever since I was a kid, I have wanted to know what was inside the body and how it worked. As a teenager, I thought I would become a doctor; part of me has always wanted to go to med school, even as an observer. As a college teacher, I have felt that texts mean the most when they link up with reality, and what's more real than the human bodies we live in? I have enjoyed authors who give some sense of the embodiment of human life—Richard Selzer, Sharon Olds, Robert Murphy, Reynolds Price, Oliver Sacks, Paul Monette, Lucy Grealy—and I wonder whether my abilities as a writer can deal with the strange sights I am about to observe. I am risking an academic year on this project, one of my rare leaves from teaching, without knowing what the results will be. In a time when granting agencies virtually want your conclusions in your proposal before any investigation, this is a strange undertaking indeed.

With excitement I push open the door to the anatomy-physiology building. I walk slowly down the hall looking for the lecture room, seeing lab-coated instructors stride briskly past me; the students, typically in shorts and carrying knapsacks, also make their way to the first class meeting.

Settling into the back of the auditorium, I take a look at these students.

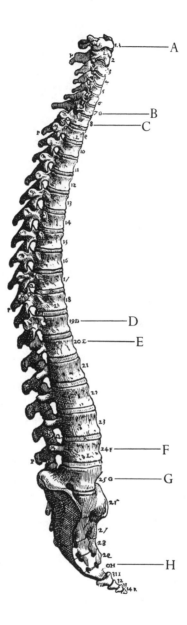

THE SPINE

(Figure 2)

From *De fabrica*, p. 57.

THE SPINE IS also known as the "vertebral column," since it is made up of vertebrae (literally, "things to turn on"). Thus the notion of "column" seems paradoxical, as if it were a central, immobile tower. Instead, however, we are fortunate enough to have both structure and flexibility in this remarkable construct.

In many Eastern traditions, the spine is identified with serpent power. In India, for example, the Kundalini is considered the vitalizing power that can rise up the spine. In the West, the staff of Asclepius and even the two-snake Caduceus (more accurately the symbol of Hermes) are other images of "serpentine healing."

The spinal cord lies within the vertebrae, sending off branches of nerves that go throughout (and return from) the body. Injuries to the cord, therefore, are usually specific; from the point of injury downward (i.e., away from the head), functions to all parts of the body are compromised.

Vesalius numbers the vertebrae from right below the head (1, or the "atlas" vertebra) to the coccyx, or 34, between the buttocks. Moderns divide the vertebrae into five categories: cervical or neck (1 through 7; "A" to "B" in the engraving), thoracic (corresponding to the twelve ribs, 8 through 19; "C" to "D"), lumbar ("of the loin": 20 through 24; "E" to "F"), and sacral (25 on down—these tend to fuse together and form joints with the two sacral bones of the pelvis). Vesalius counted six vertebrae in the sacral section ("pertaining to the sacrum"; 25; "G" to "H"), while moderns count five. The remaining vertebrae are called coccygeal ("pertaining to the coccyx," a word indicating the cuckoo bird, specifically its beak), here numbering four; moderns figure three to five; these commonly fuse as we grow up.

According to Saunders and O'Malley (page 62), Vesalius's rendition of the spinal column does a poor job with natural curves, owing to an iron bar the bones have been forcibly threaded upon.

The artist for this woodcut (and for most of the other estimated 276 of the volume) has been the subject of much debate. Many commentators have favored Jan Stefan van Kalkar, who studied with Titian (who has also been proposed as the artist). Another candidate has been Domenico Campagnola, also of Titian's studio. Some think Vesalius himself must have had a hand in some of the drawings upon which the woodcuts were made.

Over 200 of the original woodblocks survived together until World War II, when they were destroyed in the bombing of Munich.

There are 113 of them, I've been told, and they are clearly a varied lot. I see men and women, white and black, Hispanic, Asian, and Anglo, a much more diverse class than it would have been ten years ago. They are mostly in their twenties, but some are a bit older. Among the men, I see a yarmulke, a turban, and two baseball caps. There is no headgear among the women, but a profusion of black, blond, and brown hair. We take our places in rows in the traditional steep rise of medical auditoriums, so that we look down on the lecturer. In the past, this arrangement allowed viewers to peer into the body of a cadaver as it was being dissected. Today, dissecting takes place in other rooms, while the high front wall here provides a huge area for projection of slides, one at a time or two side by side, at the eye level of the audience.

The first lecture describes the aims of the course and its organization. Dr. Arthur English, the course director, clips on a microphone and explains the details. A Ph.D. in anatomy, he is a moderately tall man, with a vivid white mustache. Having taught this course many times, he explains convincingly how it works. The course has three lectures per week describing the areas of the body to be dissected in the lab: the first lecture will discuss the back, and the assignments for the first two lab sessions will be to locate the parts just described.

English then introduces the university chaplain, Donald G. Shockley, saying that he will come to the labs and be "available for anyone to talk with." English says that we should be aware that the cadavers were living persons, all of whom died in the past year. They have willed their bodies to the university for research and education. While the six members of the teaching staff always wear lab coats, Chaplain Shockley never does: in his sport coat and tie, he's a reminder of the outside, nonmedical world, and the still larger world of spirit, transcendence, and ultimate values.

"Nine years ago," Shockley says in his soft Alabama accent, "some med students came to me and said, 'It just doesn't seem right to walk away from the table without some kind of closure.' I helped them create a Service of Reflection and Gratitude, as we called it, and every class since then has carried on this tradition. Near the middle of the course, I will ask for volunteers to develop this year's service."

I have heard about this ceremony; indeed, it is one of the reasons I have come to Emory. I want to see what impact it makes on the emotions and meanings evoked by the lab two floors above us.

The next day is the first formal lecture of the course, and our topic is "The Vertebral Column and the Spine." As I listen, I imagine that students must be thinking, *How does the picture on the screen compare to the cadaver I am going to meet in the next hour?* The lecturer is Dr. Steven L. Wolf, an intense man who strides about the stage, gesturing at the huge images above him. He uses a laser pointer—a bright red arrow—to focus our attention on particular features of the slides.

The lecture over, students head up to the lab. Some take the stairs, others the elevator. The eager ones surge ahead, the reluctant ones hang back. As I enter the third-floor hallway, I smell the sharp odor of formaldehyde. Students mill around in the hallway, clustering in prearranged groups of six and checking and rechecking the bulletin board where their assignments are posted. This information includes the table numbers, with groups of six students, whose names are followed by A, B, or C to indicate the pairs, or "teams," that will dissect together. Students recheck these assignments, in part to be sure where they're going, but also, it seems to me, to delay crossing the threshold through the wooden door with the opaque window. They plop their backpacks on large metal tablelike structures in the hall (probably unaware that these embalming tanks, called New Yorkers, have a cadaver floating inside). They put on their lab coats, most of which are fresh from the store, stiff and creased in rectilinear patterns. They take books and dissecting kits in hand, push open the door, and in a mild parody of a dinner party look for the numbered tables where they will work for the next sixteen weeks. I enter too, in the borrowed lab coat that gives me protective coloration. I intend to be invisible, a mute observer hidden by a magical one-way mirror. Dr. English has told me that he'll try to find some students I can follow through the course, but today will be a more general overview.

In the three main dissecting rooms, six stainless-steel tables are arranged and numbered as shown in Figure 3. The strange numbering system, I'll learn later, is for sequencing in lab exams. There is also a fourth room, with

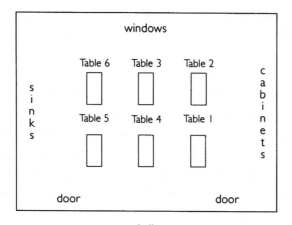

windows

	Table 6	Table 3	Table 2	
s				c
i				a
n				b
k	Table 5	Table 4	Table 1	i
s				n
				e
				t
				s

door   door

hall

FLOOR PLAN OF ANATOMY LAB

(Figure 3)

a single dissecting table, an addition caused by the large size of this year's class.

I survey one room. Each of the six tables supports a horizontal corpse wrapped in white plastic. Despite the covering, outlines of bodies are clearly discernible: the feet stick up, and the head has the necessary roundness.

I drift along the side, by the sinks. Nearby is Chaplain Shockley in his sport coat. One student passes by us and blurts out, "I don't want to touch the thing!" He doesn't stop walking, though, doesn't even look at Shockley, but continues through the tables until he finds his number.

The thirty-six students are now assembled at their tables, making a crowded room. Ordinarily, only two per table will dissect at a time, passing on their knowledge to the other four; this way a single cadaver serves six students.

The tables have solid rails all around, so that the bodies can't roll off. One end is tilted downward so that any liquids can drain into a bucket suspended under a hole. Each table has two blocks of wood to prop up parts of the body for easier exploration, and four attachments for book racks so that texts can be kept near at hand. Near each table is a big lamp on a tall, wheeled stand. There are also some twenty wheeled stools throughout the room, with circular seats of red, blue, yellow, and ivory, the only bright colors in this stark concrete room with beige walls.

There is a particular strategy at work here: by leaving the cadavers on their backs, the anatomy instructors make sure that students will have to touch and handle the dead body; the teams must work together to turn the cadaver over for the first dissection, the back. The students, therefore, will have to confront this cadaver, work as a team, and, symbolically, take charge of this dead body.

"How did he die?" I hear murmured at a nearby table.

"It's on the wall, over there, for each one," a student murmurs. I sidle over to the piece of paper taped by the door and see typed information about the cadavers; for Table 3, for example, it looks like this:

Table	Number	Sex	Age	Date of Death	Cause of Death
3	64983	F	101	AUG. 10	CVA

The five-digit number (also on a plastic band on the cadaver's wrist) will allow the university to return ashes to the family upon request. The cause of death was in this case cerebrovascular accident—probably a stroke. As I look over all the sheets I see that heart attacks, vascular disease, and cancer are the most common causes of death for these cadavers, as they are for the American population as a whole.

The class is subdued today. If students talk at all, it's very quietly and at their own tables.

The students open their boxes of latex gloves and awkwardly put them on. (Even recently, med students didn't use gloves for dissections; in the era of AIDS, however, gloves have become standard.) They draw the large white plastic sheet from the body and fold it up. Some hesitate with the damp, white blanket below, but that, too, is pulled away, and a strange sight lies there, an embalmed corpse. It seems a paradox. On the one hand, it is clearly the remains of an elderly person, a known entity. On the other hand, it is an eerie, almost unearthly version of a living body, something that is so foreign that I instinctively feel *something here is wrong, dangerous.*

As the coverings come off, the smell of formaldehyde intensifies, filling the lab.

"Nasty."

"Gross."

Students wrinkle their noses and shake their heads. Some wipe their eyes, which are running in reaction to the fumes. Others wear face masks (with activated charcoal) over their noses and mouths to lessen the fumes' effect. The syllabus warns them not to wear contact lenses in the lab because these might absorb gases and chemical irritants.

"I wish I hadn't eaten lunch," mutters one, but no one becomes sick, and no one faints this year. Fainting is rare, actually, and is often attributable to other causes, such as no food for twenty-four hours. I have heard that some students cry upon receiving their cadaver, but I don't see any tears today. Either they are hidden from me, or the emotional preparation (including the presence of the chaplain) has, somehow, been sufficient.

The cadavers themselves are a tannish gray, lacking the enlivening pink from the red cells in circulating blood. Lips and nipples are not crimson, purple, or even pink, but muddy shades of gray. The eyes are shut, the features slightly swollen, perhaps from embalming. Fingernails are grayish yellow. The nail beds underneath are gray. The hands are lightly curved, as in life. The pubic hair is generally sparse and typically without any white hairs. The hair on the head has been close-cropped on all cadavers, leaving a stubble usually gray or white. The prevalence of cadaveric white hair seems to say, *Yes, I was old enough to die; my death makes some kind of sense.*

If I look at these aged heads alone, I find that the short hair makes discerning male and female difficult. And, lying down, the cadavers give few clues to relative height. The breasts and genitalia are the obvious marks of male and female. Three long cuts are common, the work of the embalmer: one at the throat, two at the groin; these have been sewn shut in large, even stitches.

The cadavers range in age from 57 to 101. This is a comforting fact: what a horror it would be to turn back the coverings and find a young person, or one the same age as the students. There are stories that circulate about this unveiling; some seem to be folkloric renderings of our deepest fears: "Did you hear about the med student who pulled back the shroud and found her grandmother—who had just died?"

The students don't pause to observe much detail about these cadavers today. At every table they seem anxious to get the body turned over and covered up again. Doctors often say, "Yes, I remember my cadaver from med school vividly. The most emotionally difficult part for me was the face." Or, I have also heard, the hands. The students tell me later that they wanted, through draping, to make the cadaver a biological exhibit only, much like the fetal pig or shark they dissected in college.

Turning cadavers is awkward with a noncooperating subject. For some students, touching the corpse is "no big deal." Others touch gingerly. Some touch as little as possible—or even not at all. One way or the other, the groups do what the lab instructors intend: they pull the body to one side of the dissecting table and tip it up and, finally, over. Aware that this was once a person, they show respect by preventing the body from thumping over, with fair success. Some of the corpses, however, make noise on the metal as a knee, a shoulder, or a head bumps down. The chin rests on a block of wood. This prop helps depersonalize the cadaver further; clearly it is not a pillow.

The feel of embalmed flesh (I will learn next week) is strange: slightly rubbery, slightly swollen, exactly room temperature—neither warm nor cold. There is no rigor mortis, a temporary stiffness that begins a few hours after death and then diminishes with time, and the limbs flop somewhat. Arm, wrist, and hand fall to the side in the general shape of a living limb. One by one, all the cadavers are turned over. To a newcomer, it is in some ways a macabre scene, with grunts of students, flailings of dead limbs, and called-out directions. And yet, there is a mood of practicality, a purposefulness about a necessary job.

"Get that hand back on the table."

"Uncross those feet."

"Cover that head back up, will you?"

And yet, as the students work with the cadavers, they make discoveries.

"He was tan: see where the watch was?"

"He wore a wedding ring; look at the indentation."

"Her spine is twisted. What do you call that? Scoliosis?"

"This guy is really wasted away. What did he die from?"

At all tables, Team A prepares to cut into the back. Some of the other teams members stay to watch, while others leave—some rather quickly.

The student who spoke to the chaplain about his fear speaks to him again on his way out; not a Team A person, he'll make his first cut later.

"I did it! I actually touched the cadaver!" he says sidelong to Chaplain Shockley, again not breaking his stride. (I talk to him weeks later: he says he was nervous and scared that first day, glad that he didn't faint and glad to get out of the lab.)

The young and alive accept the gift of these bodies. While they certainly are not patients, they are the first bodies entrusted to the continuing care of these students for exploration, intimacy, and discovery.

THE FIRST CUT

· · ·

WHOA! . . . BETTER TURN it over so you don't cut yourself," I hear from a nearby table. The students, awkward in their gloves, are trying to put scalpel blades onto the blade holders. They have opened their brown plastic dissecting kits to take out their new tools. There are two pairs of forceps, a probe, two pairs of scissors, and, of course, the scalpel. The modern scalpel is only a metallic stick; it needs blades in order to cut. Like working surgeons, the students must have fresh blades; these blades for the anatomy lab, however, are marked "nonsterile": cadavers have no risk for infection. Except for the scalpel, most of these tools are barely changed from the Renaissance, when modern anatomy emerged as a discipline. Perhaps improvement can only come in minor variations (such as metal alloys) or entirely new instruments, such as the electrocautery (an electric probe that coagulates blood vessels while it cuts), but these students are linked by their tools to their forebears in the professions of anatomy and medicine.

"Yeah . . . if anybody's going to get cut up here, it had better be, um, them," a beginning blade fitter replies, gesturing at the prone cadaver. The bare back is pale under the fluorescent lights, while the head and lower body are draped in the soggy white blanket.

"Well, what do we have to do?"

Students throughout the room refer to the description in *Grant's*

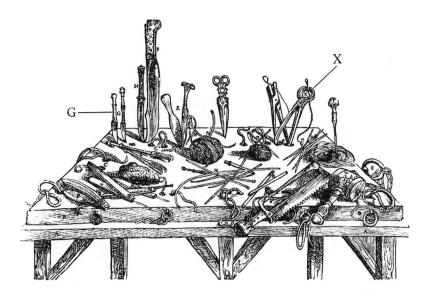

DISSECTING TOOLS

(Figure 4)

From *De fabrica,* page 235.

VESALIUS WRITES THAT all of his dissections were done with these tools. Many of them are little changed from his day: the mallet and saw (at right), for example, even the precursor to the modern rongeur (back, right, with an "x" in the opening), as well as scissors and string. The Renaissance scalpels are in one piece (back left, labeled "G"); Vesalius called them *cultelli,* or knives.

Dissector, open on a book stand like a piece of music ready to be played. The text tells the students to cut from the base of the skull, down the spine, to below the waist (to the level of the posterior superior iliac spines—the hip bones just below the small of the back). In other words, this opening cut is some two feet long.

"Do you want to do it?"

"Naaa, go ahead."

"Okay, here goes."

The scalpel moves with surprising ease. Bending close over the cadavers, the students hold the scalpel "like a cello bow," in the traditional phrase, and pull it across the skin, straight down the spine. The instrument seems to perform more like a paintbrush than a knife. The first cuts I see are shallow, tentative nicks. When no one cries out, when nothing explodes, when the heavens do not fall, students make the next cut deeper and longer, maybe eight or ten inches straight down the spine. Back skin is some of the thickest skin of the body, along with the palms of the hands and the soles of the feet, but it's no more than an eighth of an inch thick. Although it feels tough, it cuts readily, and the fat below offers no resistance to these terrifically sharp blades.

The cuts themselves are bloodless, since embalming has removed the blood from the cadavers. With repeated, bolder cuts in the same groove, the skin is fully cut, and yellow or even gold fat appears beneath, in globular cells.

In his book *Mortal Lessons,* surgeon-writer Richard Selzer has written of the scalpel: "Without the blade, the handle has a blind, decapitated look. It is helpless as a trussed maniac. But slide on the blade, click it home, and the knife springs instantly to life. It is headed now, edgy, leaping to mount fingers for a gallop to its feast." In today's lab, these beginning cutters probably don't feel the same emotions as Selzer, a veteran surgeon, but I imagine they feel other kinds of intensity. *Am I doing this right? Will I spoil my cadaver? Will I find all the structures needed for the presentation?*

The room is very quiet.

Next, four horizontal cuts transect the first vertical line, and students pull up the skin at the resultant corners, cutting it away from the fat below, "reflecting it," in the anatomical phrase. Directed by the *Dissector,* some make a "buttonhole," an inch-long cut in the pulled-up skin, so that a finger may be inserted for pulling; skin has a good tensile strength and doesn't tear readily. The fat underneath ("subdermal" or "subcutaneous") varies from corpse to corpse in color (from a light straw color to a strong yellow, almost gold—particularly in some of the women) and in amount. In life (at a higher temperature), it would be more viscous and easier to work with. Here it is more solid, although not as hard as the fat on a refrigerated steak.

Typically, women have more subdermal fat, but there is wide individual variation. At Table 4, a man has virtually no fat at all (the students will call him the Fatless Man); he's easy to cut open in one sense, but treacherous in another, since some structures are harder to find, and still others, such as superficial nerves, are easily destroyed, tearing off with the skin. At Table 6, on the other hand, a huge male cadaver is packed with fat, a full inch of it beneath the skin on his back. He immediately gains some renown in this room: "Did you see the hulk over there?" I hear more than once.

Kathy, one of the students cutting at this table, says, "Yep, he's big. We're kind of proud of him. We're going to call him Nero," she says, patting the meaty volume of his shoulder. With her brown hair in a pageboy, she looks like the girl next door, not someone about to lay open a back with a knife.

The cutting and trimming is very slow today. The students are beginners, wary of errors. They ask many questions of the instructors, waiting until one is free. As they talk quietly among themselves, a common phrase is, "Are we supposed to . . . ?" while "You got me!" is a common response.

Slowly, the students turn the skin back and "pick the fat" down to the fascia covering the muscles; this tedious task is important because it makes visible important structures, such as muscles, blood vessels, and nerves. While a lot of the fat stays with the skin flaps, students put what they remove totally into the bucket at the foot of the table. Next, they cut through the layer of plastic wrap–looking fascia covering the musculature and begin to separate muscles. They start with the outer or "superficial" muscles of the back, the trapezius, the latissimus dorsi, and other, smaller muscles. Since the aim of dissection is to define bodily structures into clarity—and not destruction—the students cut the ends of the muscles closest to the spine, but leave the other ends attached. These muscles are surprisingly thin, more like straps than the bulging structures displayed by weightlifters. (See Figure 5.)

I'm surprised by these slender muscles and wonder why. Perhaps it's because I think of muscles as part of male display, as in bodybuilding competitions or the exaggerated breastplates worn by Roman warriors—regardless of whatever wine bellies sagged behind the metal. That night I look up "muscle" in the dictionary and learn that the origin is the Latin *musculus,* for "little mouse," as if these active, wiggly things ran around under our skin. Mousles indeed!

But do moderns know much better? Unless we pay some attention to anatomy, our knowledge of muscles is, literally, superficial: we know the names of some of the exterior muscles, like the biceps, but not the underlying (or "deep," as anatomists say) muscles that are equally important. In sum, about 600 named muscles make our bodies move by bending some 200 joints. Other unnamed and uncountable smooth-muscle fibers do other jobs, such as slowly squeezing food along the intestines or quickly compressing blood vessels so that we don't faint when we stand up.

I look at the legs of nearby students. Since most are in shorts, their bare legs stick out below their lab coats as if from short skirts. The men's muscled and hairy legs look strange in this garb; the women's legs, shaved and plumped with subdermal fat, signal their sex. What evolutionary rules decreed that men would display muscle and women would display fat? Women have the same number of muscles as men, but their strength is harder to gauge visually, since women's muscles tend not to bulk up from heavy use. I once watched a woman perform ten chin-ups to the top of a door frame, gripping the narrow molding with only her fingertips. She collected a large bet from several muscular men before explaining that she was a veteran rock climber.

The talk today is quiet and serious. Perhaps Chaplain Shockley's presence makes a difference. Shockley moves through the labs, sometimes just leaning against the wall, making himself accessible. Through his horn-rimmed glasses, his blue eyes seem kind.

Seeing that no students are talking to him now, I saunter over. We've met before, so I feel free to ask him about his work.

"How's business?" I ask.

"Pretty quiet," he says.

"When students do come to you, what do they say?"

"Well, it all depends, but they might say something like, 'I wonder if I could talk to you a moment. I'm having trouble with my cadaver. You see, my grandfather died this summer.' "

"And what do you say?"

"Oh, something like, 'I understand what you mean. That must be hard. Would you like to talk about it more?' "

"And do they?"

"Sometimes . . . but often just a brief conversation seems to give the emotional release they can't find anywhere else."

I go back to my perch on a stool in the corner to watch the room as a whole, still acting the role of fly on the wall—or maybe even of some kind of dunce. I am tiring of this distant position and am eager to learn which of the nineteen tables will be "mine," which of these students I will get to know. When I spoke to Dr. English today, he told me the names of two men whom he would ask for permission. I look in my notepad and find the names, Jonathan and Steve. I wonder if they will agree to my intrusion.

The entire back will not be dissected in detail, since the emphasis in this dissection is on the vertebral column. After getting a good overview, the students are to focus on one section of the spinal column, cutting their way down to that. The *Dissector* gives the full approach, but the course syllabus lists only five learning objectives (specifically, the vertebrae, spinal musculature, the ligaments between vertebrae, the spinal nerves coming from the spinal cord, and the meninges covering the spinal cord). The students puzzle about how to dissect for these goals and realize that "one deep hole" is the answer, an excavation of, say, three inches by three inches beneath the flaps of skin and muscle they have already created. As they dig down, some of them aim their lights carefully into the area, while others don't even turn them on.

By 5:00 P.M., many of the students have decided that they've had enough for one day and that they will return to get down to that spine.

"How are we going to finish this, though?" one worried student asks his partner.

She looks at the schedule. "I don't know. We've only got three hours next Tuesday. Then we present on Thursday."

"No way . . . we need more time!"

They ask a lab instructor and learn that the lab can be used at other times, if a key is checked out. Thus the common call as we near five o'clock will become, "Who's got the key for tonight?"

In a matter of hours the first lab session, the first touching, the first incision—all these are history. The students are still beginners, but Team A has begun to dissect or, as the students say, to *cut*.

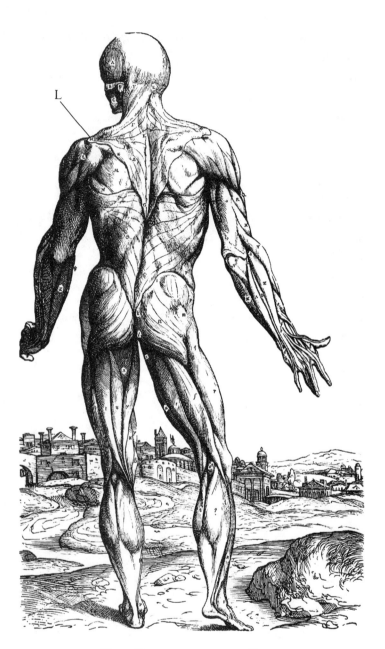

THE MUSCLES OF THE BACK

(Figure 5)

From *De fabrica*, The Ninth Plate of the Muscles, page 194.

THIS IS THE ninth plate in a series commonly called the "musclemen." The figure, shown front and back, is progressively dissected, deeper and deeper as the plates proceed. This is a highly idealized figure, of course, as if all skin, fat, superficial blood vessels, and fascia (muscle covering) could be removed—as if such a figure could stand up by itself.

Further, the figure is placed in a countryside, as if part of nature, not lying down in some charnel house. The human body, even as a cadaver for dissection, thus seems natural and powerful.

If the musclemen woodcuts are placed side by side, the backgrounds form (at least in theory) a continuous scene. Harvey Cushing identified the locale as being near Abano Terme in the Euganean Hills, southwest of Padua, where old Roman baths ("terme") lie in ruins, according to Saunders and O'Malley (page 29).

The Renaissance stylization gives the figure (and the landscape) elegance and clarity. The cross-hatching that shades this woodcut gives texture and a sense of modeling, or roundness. The shadow from the left leg on the ground and the shadowed left arm imply that the source of light, presumably the sun, is from the right. Viewing the figure from such a low angle gives it an air of monumentality.

The multitude of symbols (largely Roman and Greek letters) that spangle the figure help Vesalius's text identify the names of the muscles. "L" on the shoulder, for example, indicates the deltoid muscle, frequently the site, in modern times, for hypodermic injections.

CAN YOU GIVE US
A HAND HERE?

• • •

THE FIRST DEAD body I remember seeing was a cadaver on a university campus. I was in seventh grade, taking an art course in a multipurpose building. As we zoomed around before school, one kid ran up, bug-eyed, and hissed, "There's a dead man upstairs!"

"Naw . . . you're putting me on . . . where?"

We crept upstairs to a room that was evidently part of some lab. Holding our breaths against the smell, we peeked around the door frame to see a cadaver on a table, naked except for a towel over chest and groin.

A series of dares and pushes advanced us toward the table. I lifted a corner of the towel enough to see the layers of exposed musculature. Then our bravado collapsed and we ran like hell.

Shortly we were in class, glad we were not in trouble. We did not go up those stairs again nor even mention that strange event. I haven't told anyone about this until now.

As schoolkids in our culture, we were entirely unprepared to view such a sight. It is a rarity to see a dead person in America, except at funerals, where clothing and cosmetics normally cover the body. As the anatomy course proceeds, I learn that many of the students have scant experience with dead bodies; some have never seen one until the first day of lab. For better or worse, the anatomy course is a crash course in death: you can't spend sixteen weeks with nineteen cadavers without feeling and pondering death. Much has been written about the American aversion to our dead, our strange funeral practices, and the general disappearance of the cadaver from the mourners' attention. In many cultures (and in some American subcultures) it is the custom for family to bathe and dress the cadaver, to hold a wake with the dead body on, say, the dining room table, to make the coffin and dig the grave, to lower the coffin into the grave. I remember serving as a pallbearer for Jan, a woman I had loved in my college years. Some twenty years later she died of cancer. I visited her in her final weeks, then felt the heavy weight of her casket through the metal ring in my hand. While this weight was welcome—and healing to me—I wish I could have done more for her. In some ways death has been stolen from us, and we no longer have ways of understanding it personally and practically. This ignorance makes us all the more vulnerable to misunderstanding, fears, and even terror. Because physicians and clergy are among the few still knowledgeable about death, we place on them a tremendous responsibility to deal with it in our stead. When physicians fail to protect us from death, we feel betrayed. I wonder whether this morass of ignorance, fear, and betrayal is one source of the dramatic increase of medical malpractice suits. In my own experience with my father dying of cancer, my family and I were not ready for many events and emotions that were thrust upon us. Our trials came before the hospice movement in America, which serves terminally ill patients and their families in their last six months of life with advice, comfort, understanding of pain relief, and the like.

"Where'd you get that?" I ask one student, pointing to a set of cleaned vertebrae on a circle of string. It looks like an oversized necklace. Quite oversized, really: the bones are big because they are human. He explains that each team has checked out a "bone box" with a set of disarticulated human bones for study at home or, in this case, for use in a presentation. This is news to me, the notion that you can check out someone's bones, just like a book.

Today is the second lab for Team A, the day when they should finish their dissection of the back and start to prepare their presentations. On my way to the lab Dr. English catches me in the hall and tells me that Jonathan and

Steve have agreed to let me observe at their table when they—as Team B—begin to work on the next lab.

Since I have no wish to sit in the corner today, I wander around all four rooms. The tables are similar, with two or three lab-coated students bending over the opened back of their cadaver. In every case the rest of the body is thoroughly covered up.

"Can you give us a hand here?" one group asks me, somewhat to my alarm: I was hoping to be a perceiver just drifting by. These two students, a man and a woman, are deep into the back. In my professional-looking lab coat, I am reasonably mistaken for one of the instructors. "Nope, I'm sorry. I'm an observer," I confess, truly sorry I can't help these students—ordinarily my role in life, but not here.

"I'm not an anatomist," I explain. There's an awkward pause and they stare at me. "I'm a humanist, observing your course, hoping to write something about it."

"Oh," one says.

No one knows what to say next, and I wander on.

SIR WILLIAM HARVEY
PINCH-HITS
• • •

ECTURE DAY. I settle into the back of the auditorium as usual, sitting with the instructors in the last row. Several faculty remark to me, "This will probably be the best lecture of the year!"

Thus I am surprised when Art English takes the podium and looks apologetic.

"I'm sorry," he intones, "to have to make this announcement about this morning's lecture, particularly since we take pride in the organization of this course, as complex as it is, but I got a phone call this morning—that the lecturer couldn't make it."

Students look at each other. I feel genuine disappointment, since the announced topic, "The Functional Anatomy of the Heart," should be fascinating. "The message was," Dr. English persists, "that Dr. Silverman's athlete's foot was acting up terribly, but that he had found a substitute."

Now wait a minute—lots of heads are turning around, as if to ask: *Is English on the level?*

"And when I interviewed this substitute, it appeared to me that he would be up to the task. Actually he knows a lot about it: please welcome Sir William Harvey!"

Baroque music wells up from the projection booth and "Sir William" walks majestically down the middle aisle. He is dressed in a seventeenth-century costume, with a large, floppy white collar and a multicolored

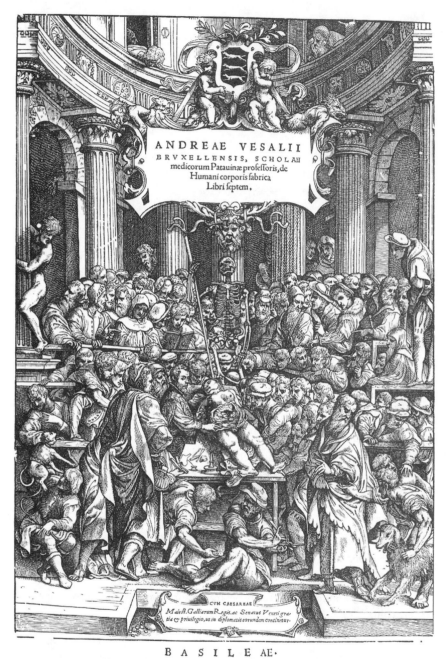

ANDREAE VESALII
BRVXELLENSIS, SCHOLAE
medicorum Patauinæ professoris, de
Humani corporis fabrica
Libri septem.

CVM CAESAREAE
Maiest.GalliarumR.egis, ac Senatus Veneti gra-
tia & priuilegio, ut in diplomatis eorundem continetur.

BASILEAE·

TITLE PAGE, *DE HUMANI CORPORIS FABRICA*

(Figure 6)

IN THE ELABORATE style of early printed books, this large woodcut is packed with detail. (The following comments owe heavily to Saunders and O'Malley, page 42.)

The scene is a public anatomy demonstration by Vesalius, the bearded figure just to the left of the (female) cadaver, the only person clearly touching it. Breaking with tradition, he does the work himself, placing the "menials" below the table, where they quarrel. His tools and a candle are on the corner of the table. (In the second edition, a pen in an ink pot and a paper with writing join the scene.)

The demonstration is outside (see greenery in the arch at the left), before an ornate Palladian building. A temporary wooden platform supports the guests, students, and fellow physicians, as well as leaders of the city and the Church.

The monkey and the dog represent Galen's dependence on animal dissections; rejected by Vesalius, these are far from the center. Indeed, a robed, bearded figure between the dog and the cadaver admonishes the dog, hand upraised.

The articulated skeleton in the center suggests the importance of understanding the underlying bones, while the nude figure to the left symbolizes surface anatomy, particularly in living action—note the dynamic pose. (In the second edition, the figure to the left is clothed and the staff held by the skeleton becomes a scythe of death.)

The shield at the top shows three weasels running, "the crest of Vesalius, and a play on the vernacular version of his name, Wessels," in Saunders and O'Malley's phrase.

doublet. He carries a huge tome in his hand, presumably his revolutionary book on the heart, *De motu cordis et sanguinis in animalibus (On the Motion of the Heart and Blood in Animals)*.

Our lecturer (Mark E. Silverman, M.D.) assumes the podium and formally begins, "My name is William Harvey and I am four hundred and eleven years old. You'd think Emory wouldn't assign someone of my stature chores in freshman Anatomy, but perhaps it's because I haven't published anything since the seventeenth century." [Laughter]

"I'm here to tell you about the most important discovery of all time, *my* discovery of the circulation of blood in the body. First slide, please."

The first slide shows a portrait of Sir William, and the accuracy of Silverman's costume is suddenly clear. Silverman strikes the same pose, and the students applaud.

He continues, telling us about Harvey's life, illustrating with slides. One is a map of Europe with a red star for Padua. "I went to Padua—a foreign medical school—not because I couldn't get into one in my own country [appreciative laughter reflects domestic/foreign conflicts in training], but because it was the best in the world, a small southeastern medical school without a football team" [uproarious laughter, as Padua, southeast in Europe according to the map, and Emory University are unexpectedly made parallel].

Silverman goes on to talk about the medical knowledge and methods of the seventeenth century, including the dominance of Galen, the Greek physician of the second century after Christ. "As it was said as late as sixteen forty-nine: 'If dissection differed from Galen, it was because nature had changed'!" It is hard for us in the twentieth century to understand such blind acceptance of authority. Aristotle became a similar model; he gave a number for human teeth in women that was incorrect—when all he had to do was look in Mrs. Aristotle's mouth to get the right answer. Empirical research wasn't his method, nor did anyone challenge him for a long time.

Galen worked with animal cadavers and the wounds of Roman gladiators, Silverman continues, and theorized that natural spirits, animal spirits, and the *pneuma*—or the vital spirit—moved around the body.

With the invention of movable type in the West (Gutenberg) and the development of accurate anatomical drawings (Da Vinci and others), the mass media were all set for the revolution of Andreas Vesalius, a native of Flanders, who had dissected animals as a kid [appreciative laughter]. As a grown man, Vesalius stole the bodies of criminals who were hanged outside of Paris, took them home and dissected them, often finding Galen to be wrong. After moving to Padua, he published *De humani corporis fabrica (The Fabric of the Human Body)* in 1543, "drawing a savage reaction from those who had bought the wrong book" [huge laughter: the students have paid over $100 for their anatomy texts alone].

The next slide is the frontispiece of *De fabrica,* as it is traditionally called. (See Figure 6 above.) The title is set into an elaborate illustration, which Silverman says is satiric: it shows a dissection in a theater, with the barber-surgeons chained underneath the table—banished from true medical dissection as "slashers"—and with animals far off to the side, to indicate their inappropriateness for understanding the human body. The book uses the woodcut illustrations heavily, almost 300 of them. Perhaps most famous is the "musclemen" series, skinned and partially dissected male bodies "in nature," not dead on a table, but standing on a hillside, for example, with muscles displayed as if in use. (See Figure 7 below.) For all this, Vesalius is regarded as the father of modern anatomy.

Silverman goes on to explain how he himself—William Harvey, that is—studied under the successors to Vesalius, returned to England, and figured out the circulation of the heart. He published his revolutionary volume, *De motu cordis* (in the short title) in 1628. Although the microscope wouldn't be developed until the eighteenth century, ultimately allowing scientists to understand the capillary link between veins and arteries, Harvey concluded in Chapter XIV that "the blood is driven into a round."

While Silverman has been speaking so far as William Harvey, he suddenly says, in a less portentous voice, "It's really hot in here," and takes off his fancy doublet and white shirt with the floppy collar. Underneath is a T-shirt with the heart and great vessels portrayed in vivid color.

"I'm not really William Harvey, but Mark Silverman, a cardiologist, and

I'd like to take you on a journey inside the heart as we understand it today, on a kind of *Fantastic Voyage*. Who starred in that?" he asks, meaning the movie, and flashes up a slide of those actors.

"Raquel Welch," a dozen male voices yell out, with conviction.

"Anyone remember the male lead?"

Silence.

"Well, for you trivia fans, it was Stephen Boyd. And what is he looking at here?" The slide shows Boyd's eyes riveted to Welch's chest. [Laughter] Silverman continues to describe the chambers, valves, and vessels of the heart. He shows an X ray of his own chest ("Isn't it nice?") and remarks that the tricuspid valves always remind him of Botticelli's "Three Graces" (shown in another slide). But there is something else.

"Please raise the screen," he says, and the enormous white screen rises slowly in front of us. It has been so constantly used that I assumed it was permanent. To have it rise majestically seems a rending of the veil. Behind we see the glass screen of a huge television built into the wall.

"Let me show you some echocardiography we did this morning." Dr. Silverman punches the controls and a videotape plays on the screen. It's a tape made by ultrasound, showing the heart many times actual size as it pumps. Furthermore, a computer process has colored the Doppler signals of the moving blood red, orange, and yellow, so that there are fluid explosions of dazzling color in the chambers and through the valves, a kind of liquid fireworks in the hypnotic rhythm of a beating heart. It is spellbinding to watch the four chambers compress and expand, the valves between them open and close.

"Jesus—he didn't have that last year," one instructor whispers. All one-hundred-plus of the audience stare, mouths agape.

"Are you amazed?" Silverman asks.

"Yes!" we say with one loud voice.

"Well, that was today, a real patient. She had some blood between the layers of her pericardium, and we had to get it out. Knowing the anatomical structures of the heart is not just a curiosity," he concludes, "but something we use to treat people. As Harvey said, 'No physiological theory can be true unless it gives a complete and final explanation of all points of structures.' And, naturally, we want to use such knowledge in medical healing."

It seems improbable, after such a fine presentation, but there are more remarks to come, and these are, for this audience, no less fascinating.

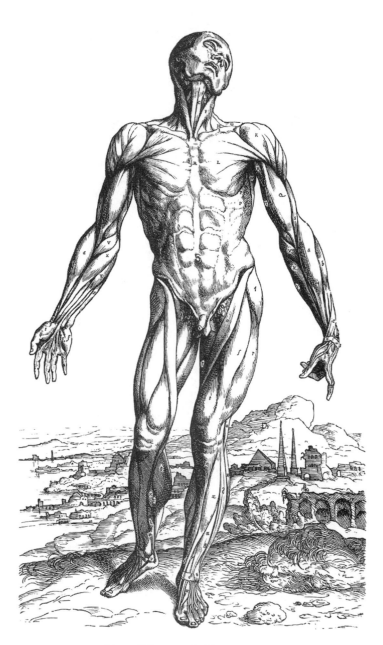

The "Flayed" Muscleman

(Figure 7)

From *De fabrica,* The First Plate of the Muscles, page 170.

IN THIS FRONT view, the muscles have been cleaned of skin, fat, blood vessels, and fascia (covering) to reveal muscles with dramatic clarity, as if the figure had been perfectly flayed. Vesalius wrote that the plate should help painters and sculptors understand superficial musculature.

Although the figure here is a well-developed man, a woman would have the same number of muscles in the same organization. While men's muscles tend to grow bigger under repeated usage, women's muscles tend not to "bulk up," even while becoming stronger.

This figure's forearms are disproportionately large, probably to display better the muscles there.

A GLIMPSE OF VESALIUS

• • •

OINING DR. SILVERMAN at the front of the room, Carol A. Burns, director of Emory's Health Sciences Library, takes five minutes to show us an original copy of Vesalius's book *De fabrica*. She also shows some slides of the detailed woodcuts and the illustrations around capital letters—some of them satirical of Renaissance anatomists. But the main fascination is the book itself, which she holds up for us, like a holy relic. This rare volume cost $500 in 1930 when professors and medical students chipped in to purchase it. Today, similar copies sell at auction for between $20,000 and $50,000, she says. Even from the back of the room, I can tell that it's physically a big book—"a real brick," as the Italians put it.

After her brief remarks, she invites students to come down from their rows and see this Vesalius up close. A large number surge forward. A book lover myself, I want to examine it in some detail, and promise myself that I will visit it in the library later. I want to touch it, to see it up close.

Physicians *see* a patient in an office; they peer into a throat or an ear, they listen to our lungs and heart, they feel for swollen lymph nodes in the neck. By such sensuous means do they perceive us, means that they have carefully learned through many years of training. I've recently learned that med students can buy a tape recording of various sounds the heart makes, in both healthy and diseased states. Clearly seeing is not just looking, but perception through a variety of the basic senses, all informed by study and practice. I'm told that a friction rub in the heart, once clearly heard, is readily heard and diagnosed at any time in the future. Similarly, a gallbladder that has been highly calcified (a "porcelain gallbladder") is so characteristic on X ray that radiologists call it (and similar findings) Aunt Minnies—you'd know her anywhere. I've been reading Michel Foucault's *Birth of the Clinic: An Archaeology of Medical Perception,* which offers the concept of "the gaze." Foucault's version of the gaze is not easily summarized, since his book is about changes in medical perception over some 200 years. Originally, of course, the gaze was basically sight, the looking at a patient, but for Foucault, it became a wider sense of an epistemology, a way of knowing. This gaze changes as philosophies, language, and institutions change. In the nineteenth century, for example, with the development of stethoscopes, the gaze became more "plurisensorial," as sight, touch, and hearing were all ways of perceiving patients. In the twentieth century, critics have argued, the patient has almost disappeared, masked by a cloud of "data," numbers churned out by machines. The MRI (magnetic resonance imager), for example, sends a radio wave into the patient and receives back another wave, which is fed to a computer that organizes the information into images of startling clarity and detail; furthermore, the image can be created in different planes, as if the body had been sliced up and down, from side to side, or from front to back.

The students rely heavily on seeing and on the cutting, which slowly reveals structures and trims them into clarity. While they ignore senses of smell and sound, they sharpen their eyes to see anatomical relationships, to learn the basic geography of the body, which will serve them during all of their professional lives. Somehow there is a conversation between touching, seeing, memorizing, reading texts, hearing lectures, thinking about everything—both for the students and for me—but it all comes back to bodies, living or dead, especially for students. For me, it all comes back to books, whether the monument of Vesalius, modern accounts, or the book I've assigned myself to write.

I FEEL LIKE A BUTCHER

· · ·

ECTURE IS OVER, and Dr. English waves to me.

"Howard, I want you to meet Steve and Jonathan."

"Great," I say, looking around.

"This is Steve Grant," English says, indicating a black-haired man with an expressive face and quick eyes. We shake hands. "And this is Jonathan Kalish," gesturing toward a tall man with curly brown hair and the white baseball cap I've seen before.

"Howard's here on leave from his college, as I told you. He wants to look over your shoulders in the lab and learn something about how you become doctors."

"That's cool," Steve says, "if you don't mind the fumes."

"Yeah, or our jokes," Jonathan puts in.

Today Team A is to present their findings to the lab instructors. Steve and Jonathan (Team B) have already heard the presentation and decide to use the time until Table 3 is open to review the objectives for dissection number two, the chest.

So we sit down in the student lounge, and they flap open their books. I'm not sure how much small talk to attempt, since I'm still thinking of myself as an observer, but I ask them about an anatomical atlas on a chair across the room.

"That's one of those colored atlases. Very expensive," Steve scoffs.

"For the real gunners," Jonathan adds, suggesting, I take it, that they are *regular* students, not candy-ass perfectionists. They don't seem to be goof-offs either, since they've already marked up their own texts with colored inks. They turn the pages perfunctorily. They seem to be on the same wavelength; later I learn that they were roommates for their undergraduate work at the University of Michigan.

"Reading doesn't really help until you get to the body," Steve says.

"Yeah," Jonathan affirms. "It's just a bunch of words, unless you can see and feel *the stuff*"—he gestures with his hand turned up, grabbing the air. The men snap their books shut. Our review of texts is at an end.

"So, why are *you* here?" Jonathan asks.

I explain that I am a humanities professor wanting to observe and hoping to write something about the anatomy lab.

"Why would anyone—of *their own free will*—choose to spend time in an anatomy class?" Jonathan asks with emphasis. He shakes his head from side to side. "I mean, we *have* to do this, but . . . you!" Steve raises his eyebrows, as if to ask the same question.

"Well, it is a bit strange," I say, "but it's a rare opportunity, really. I've always been curious about how the body works, and very few people ever get to do something like this."

They nod. "Well, maybe so. But it smells terrible up there. And wait 'til you see Little Old Lady," Jonathan warns me. *What can he mean?* I wonder.

Soon we are headed upstairs, where Team A is finishing up the presentation on the back.

"It's all yours, guys," Team A says, jubilant at having finished their assignment and, it appears, having done well. They are two men with brown hair. I don't get much more of an impression, because they are gone with the speed of light. The cadaver stays, of course, her dissected back brilliantly lit by the lamp. The flaps of skin and muscle have all been replaced, so the torso looks as though a multiple letter H has been inscribed there. Her head and lower body are covered.

"Well, I guess we have to turn her over," Steve says.

"That's the job," Jonathan grudgingly concurs.

The men slowly turn the cadaver over. The woman's body may be some 100 years old, but it is still solid, stocky even. The word *durable* doesn't seem adequate; perhaps something more like *imposing* would be better. It's not that she's so large—five-four or five-five—perhaps 110 pounds. But, still, there's something weighty beyond the actual poundage. She is an object to handle with care: 101 years old, born before the turn of this century. She could have been the great-grandmother of the men who are about to open her chest.

"Oh, that's harsh—look at her face," Jonathan says. It is the face of an old woman, surely a face that has seen much. Her mouth and eyes seem swollen. Her nose is flattened and pushed to one side, owing to the weight of her head on it during the dissection of her back.

Steve and Jonathan cover her face and lower body so that only the chest remains uncovered. The flat breasts hang to the side, with their gray nipples pointing outward. The men study the diagram in the book, which shows the seven incisions that will lay her chest open. They aim the light carefully and put blades on their scalpels. They move to opposite sides of the table, ready to make their first cuts.

"Well, let's do it," says Jonathan.

"Here we go, ready or not," says Steve. I'm glad it's them cutting and not me.

As with the back, the dissectors make the prescribed cuts, tentative at first, then with more authority. Steve and Jonathan learn how to cut under the corners of the skin, so that flaps can be pulled back. Next they trim away the underlying fat—a half inch of it—down to the fascia, the covering of the muscles. It is slow, slow work. Eventually, Steve finds a delicate structure buried in her subcutaneous fat, a white sprig like a stiff thread.

"Must be an *anterior cutaneous twig,*" Steve deliberately says of the nerve structure. "Hey, we actually found something!"

"Pretty good for two clueless cutters," Jonathan says, snipping away on his side of the table. He seems discouraged, maybe even disgusted.

"We'd better *appreciate* it," Steve says, parodying the medical use of that word. There seems to be an unwritten but general rule in medicine that multisyllabic words have more force than simple ones. It's generally better to "visualize" than to "see," better to "obliterate" than to "cut," better to have "adjuvant therapy" than "other treatment."

"I'm appreciating it," Jonathan assures him.

"Good. I'd say we appreciated the hell out of it."

They cut onward, deeper. After about an hour flaps and the underlying fat are pulled back from the sternum (breastbone). These flaps hang at the sides down to the table, carrying one breast to each side. In this dissection the breasts are not opened; their contents would be almost all fat, especially in an elderly woman, whose mammary glands would largely have atrophied.

"Remember Quincy—on the TV show?" Jonathan asks.

"Yeah."

"Just like this, everywhere he went, a whole bunch of problems."

"But he solved his," Steve says.

"And was a *hero.*" Jonathan frowns.

Steve and Jonathan cut and snip. It is very slow. They seem depressed at the lack of progress. Other students feel the same. "I almost went to law school," one passerby says. "Maybe I should have!"

"I feel like a butcher," Jonathan says, shaking his head. "I hate this place."

This is a short day, with time already taken out for the Team A presentations. Steve and Jonathan don't get very far by five o'clock and make plans to meet again, despite the immediate prospect of the Labor Day weekend. Using a plastic shaker bottle of preservative liquid (phenoxyethanol), they sprinkle the body, much as people sprinkle laundry to keep it moist for ironing. Then they cover the body carefully.

The preservative fights mold in the cadavers, one of the ways our bodily elements recycle into the ecosystem. In the anatomy lab, the cadavers take an artificial rest in their trajectory toward reincorporation into the earth.

Walking home that evening, I think about Jonathan's question: why am I up in the lab? Am I crazy to spend a semester in that grim place, off limits to normal people? What does this make me, some kind of intruder or voyeur? Am I just teasing myself about becoming a doctor? Steve and Jonathan—*real* med students—don't even like the place. Why should I?

I walk through Lullwater Park, a hilly, forested tract. Birds flit among the trees. I can smell the bosky odors of leaves decaying on the red clay. Death and life are intertwined here—and in the anatomy lab. It's not my fault that society is so aversive about death. I will claim the right to know about bodies after death, to find out whether dissection is an extremity of human experience or closer to its center. "Nothing human is alien to me," said the old Roman Terrence.

I think once again of my father, dead some twenty years. The summer I was hoping to complete my Ph.D. dissertation, I went home to nurse him and to help my mother, a thousand miles away from my wife. Dad had cancer of the brain, a glioblastoma, a diffuse growth that could be only partly removed by surgery and only partly relieved by radiation. As a family, we knew he was doomed and made the best of it. We didn't know how long he'd live in his feeble and drugged state; one doctor said ten years—a notion that scared us. When it was time for me to take up my first teaching job, I reluctantly left him. Even though my mother and I were in touch by phone, his death about two months later was a terrible blow, for many reasons. I came back for the funeral and all the difficult chores, but I never saw his body, which was prepared by a mortician and sent to a state medical school. Would my mourning have been easier if I had seen him dead? My understanding of his body on its journey was vague and unsatisfying. What happened to his body at the med school? Did the students do right by him?

A CADAVER NOW

· · ·

THE LECTURE TUESDAY is on the cardiovascular and lymphatic systems. I sit in the lecture hall and take notes, but I am eager to see how the dissection of the chest has progressed upstairs. I meet Jonathan and Steve after the lecture.

"How's it going?" I ask.

"Oh, great. We spent *seven hours* in the lab over the Labor Day weekend. *Labor* Day—what a joke! The worst Labor Day of my life. How was your Labor Day?" Jonathan asks.

"I'm embarrassed to say how nice it was; a picnic and everything."

"Well, I'm glad *someone* had a good time. But we found all sorts of stuff. Wait 'til you see the lungs!"

The guys are so excited I can hardly believe it's the same fellows who considered themselves "clueless" four days earlier. We make the obvious jokes about "labor" and "laboratory" as we make our way up the stairs, two at a time.

The men uncover the cadaver. It looks, initially, much the same, since the chest flaps have been folded back to their original positions. Thus the torso is crossed by several neat, symmetrical cuts.

"Okay, check this out." Steve and Jonathan turn back the skin flaps and identify structures.

"This is the pectoralis major muscle"—they pull the large flaps of mus-

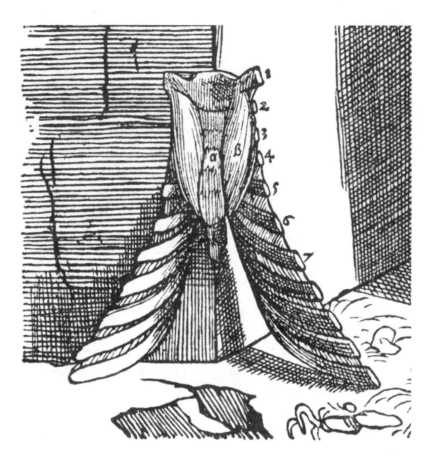

THE RIB PLATE

(Figure 8)

From *De fabrica*, detail of The Eighth Plate of the Muscles, page 192.

THIS IS A RIB plate, the section of the bone from the front of the chest. The central part is the breastbone (sternum), from which the ribs fan out on their way around to the thoracic vertebrae of the spine.

The modern rib plate is usually cut much smaller, closer to the sternum.

cle up over the shoulder—"and the underlying pectoralis minor." They pull up the two thinner muscles and clip these to the first muscle with hemostats—a very professional touch. (These are the famous "pecs" of the weight room, the chest muscles that pull the upper arms toward each other; I'd guess that these men used to say "pec," but will now use the full anatomical name, at least up here in the lab.)

As they show me the structures, a small crowd of fellow students gathers. Not many of them have gotten as far as Steve and Jonathan, who are suddenly guides for the others. They pull off the sternum (the breastbone) with a small fan of ribs to each side, all neatly cut out. This is called the rib plate; you can see it in one of the woodcuts in Vesalius. (See Figure 8.)

"Hey, you guys really got in there!" another student says.

"Yep, but there's lots more to do. Look at these lungs, though." They pull a plastic bag (from the bookstore) from under the sheets and take out two purplish objects, somewhat stiffer than in life. The lungs are light and spongy, permeated by millions of tiny air sacs called alveoli, where gases exchange between inhaled air and the body's blood. It is commonly said that the alveoli help increase the surface of the lung to such an extent that the lungs entirely flattened out could cover a tennis court.

"And look at the heart, just standing right there!" Steve exclaims.

Inside the thoracic cavity, the heart with its surrounding tissues looks like a big knot on a cable, dividing spaces on either side, where the lungs were. I am disappointed that I missed all this cutting but quickly realize that most of the chests in the room haven't been opened yet, so I'll still see plenty of action.

"Here, have a feel," Jonathan invites me, waving a lung in my direction.

"Well . . ." I say, turning up an ungloved palm.

"Get a glove on!" he urges. So I pull on a glove from their box, wiggling my fingers into the powdered, stretchy latex.

I feel the lung, heft it, then touch the cadaver. There's a slight give to the flesh.

"Put your fingers in the heart," he says.

I feel along the sides for the severed great vessels and my forefinger slips right in. It is the thick-walled left atrium, I think, surprisingly fragile feeling, considering that it worked for just over a hundred years. I feel wonder— and a strange kind of relief at reaching such an intimate recess of the human body. And yet I think this is no ultimate discovery; the secrets of human life are beyond the mere touching of inner tissues.

Jonathan reads from the text, banging his scalpel on the page, " 'Without waste *of time,* remove additionally . . .' " He pauses and grins. "I *love* it," he says sarcastically, considering the hours already invested.

"But maybe we can still find some good stuff for Halloween," Steve exhorts.

Work continues steadily around the room. This early in the course the teams stick close to their own cadaver; as the weeks roll on, they will travel more to the other tables throughout all four rooms for comparison. Today they travel only as far as their nearest neighbors.

"Yours smells better."

"Ours is 'The Body of Oddities,' " a woman says at Table 5. Sure enough, the cadaver's scoliotic spine is severely bowed to one side. Another team will call it "Quasi," after Victor Hugo's Quasimodo, the Hunchback of Notre Dame.

"Look at these lungs—full of black stuff. We ought to show gradeschoolers these to keep them from smoking!" I hear from another table.

I ask various students whether they give their cadavers names, since this is a long tradition in anatomy courses, for example, "Nero," at Table 6. I ask Kathy about that name.

"Well, he looks like a Roman aristocrat," Kathy told me. "He certainly ate a lot of good food."

The men at Table 1 have another approach. "Oh sure, that's Rose," they say.

"How come?"

"I don't know. We just looked at her and felt that her name was Rose." In another room, two cheery women state decisively, "His name is Ebenezer."

"Why?"

"Hard to say . . . I guess we just felt we could work better with him if he had that name," she says.

Still another student has decided on Job. I ask why.

"I figure I'm going to put him through the trials of Job," he says. I wonder to what extent the trials are actually *his,* not the cadaver's.

Another young man says thoughtfully, "We didn't give her a name at all. We felt that would be condescending, since she already had one in life. Besides, we didn't want to think of her still as a person. It's a cadaver, now." In each case, the student projects the name (or lack thereof) that symbolizes a good working relationship: the naming seems to say more about the students than about the cadavers.

Nero has the pale outline of his wristwatch on his forearm. Apparently he was an active man until his heart attack at age sixty-six. The cutters at that table are aware of his past prowess. "Everything about him is big—*everything,*" they say.

I too feel an urge to use names to make order; I make a survey of the cadavers' names and match it up with the information about the students posted in the hall. Pretty soon I have a chart of all the "players" (a common medical slang term for patients) in Room 1, dead or alive. (See Figure 9.) The students are getting to know each other: as they call across the room and visit among tables, each team of twelve begins to create its own social identity. During the first few days of lab, our humanity was compromised; we were emotionally and socially paralyzed by such a strange experience. As we become more habituated to the place and to each other, webs of humanity grow from table to table, from person to person.

Back at Table 3, Steve and Jonathan peer into their open chest cavity. Their eyes move between the body and their texts, trying to match up the two.

"Where is that damn azygous vein," says Jonathan. Both men poke and probe in the chest.

CUTTERS AND CADAVERS BY TABLE

(Figure 9)

(Capital letters indicate team; numbers indicate tables.)

6	*Nero*	3	*Little Old Lady*	2	*Fred*
A	Kathy	A	David	A	Mei
A	Elizabeth	A	Cliff	A	Tassos
B	Aravind	B	Steve	B	Saeed
B	Mike	B	Jonathan	B	Tim
C	Alex	C	Lisa	C	Jenifer
C	Brad	C	Jocelyne	C	Stephen
5	*Quasi*	4	*Fatless Man*	1	*Rose*
A	Karen	A	Maggie	A	Pete
A	Konny	A	Eugene	A	Bill S.
B	Bill P.	B	Melanie	B	John
B	Keith	B	Doug	B	Larry
C	Jim	C	Karl	C	Dave
C	Margaret	C	Charlie	C	Chris

(Note: Not all students use the same name for the same cadaver. At Table 3, for example, Steven and Jonathan use "Little Old Lady," but David and Cliff prefer not to have a name.)

"Hey, that's it—*right there!*" Steve calls out. "We've been looking at it all along!"

What's happened for Steve? Obviously, he has made a connection between a bit of the body right in front of him and the technical term he is supposed to know; much of the course will continue in this vein of matching physical reality (including the relations to other structures and, of course, their function within the body) to a long list of terms. In the two levels of names—the technical anatomical lingo and the personal names for the cadavers—students are creating a working relationship with a human body. Clearly the mood of Steve and Jonathan has changed, from disgust and maybe even despair, to elation and enthusiastic involvement. They have experienced one of the rites of passage in the lab. One way or another, the students are slowly creating a functional relationship between themselves and these bodies, or, wider still, between themselves and any human bodies, dead or alive. This is no small shift in orientation; while it goes by tiny steps in the lab, it seems to me, over the long run of training, to be a heroic jump. I think of the neurosurgeon who worked on my father's brain; years later he remembered the case and said he was sorry that there was not more he could do. This meant a lot to me, since medicine can seem always successful, the complete problem solver, even, on occasion, a profession of arrogance that does not know how to deal with death.

SAWING INTO THE CHEST

· · ·

THERE ARE SEVERAL ways into a chest, varying with the purposes and the speed required. In a trauma center the phrase "to crack the chest" means to get in as quickly as possible, typically for a desperate attempt to repair some major blood vessels or massage the heart to restart it. This is a high-risk procedure: the patient is near death anyway, and quick entry offers the only (and small) chance he may have—and usually it is a male. Stabbings or gunshot wounds often cause such trauma to the chest. As an emergency room volunteer I've seen a trauma surgeon crack a chest. The patient, in extremis, had no anesthetic. The surgeon, still in his shirtsleeves, made a few quick cuts between the ribs, put in the rib spreader, and cranked them apart. With another cut, he was inside to look and, especially, to feel. The patient bled heavily; the nurses hung units of blood, five, six, eight, nine pints. "What's the blood pressure?" the surgeon asked. It was low, something like 70 over 35. It continued to drop, while the surgeon sewed up some vessels but found others shredded.

"It's no use," he finally said, dropping his tools. "The whole aortic arch is gone." Shortly the surgeon pronounced him dead, and everyone looked at the clock while a nurse wrote this information on the chart.

Talking with some of the med students, I remember the event and tell them about it. Some have witnessed similar events—while working in the medical world—but most have not. Says one, "Boy, I just hope I can think quickly enough to make the right decisions." He pauses over the tedious dissection of the intercostal muscles. "This work here is so slow!"

Across the room Kathy picks up a saw from a stack next to the sinks. A strange collection, they lie there as casually as on my tool bench at home: There's a backsaw, ordinarily for cabinetwork; a metal-handled saw, much like a pruning saw; and what I take to be an anatomical saw. These are all mottled from long use, but otherwise inexpressive of the strange work they have done over the years. *Great,* I think, *now I can see how the chest is opened.*

"Well, let's do it," Kathy's partner Elizabeth urges, and they start to cut. The saw goes back and forth across the breastbone with the familiar sound of sawing: *nernnf nernnf nernnf.* Dr. English has told me that some students have never sawed anything when they come to the lab: surely a human body would be a tough material to start on. Furthermore, I have read in the syllabus that in a few weeks, they will have to saw in half the head itself. I look at Nero's head. Saw *that* in half?

Whether these women have experience or not, they saw efficiently across Nero's chest, while he shakes and sways beneath their efforts. In a few minutes they are through the sternum. They size up the ribs on either side and test how the saw can fit. The angle is hard, especially on a large chest, but they reach over his shoulders to make two vertical cuts, sawing through the ribs in short order. Even on someone as large as Nero, ribs aren't very thick. Eventually all bones are separated by hand from the underlying tissues, and they pull off the rib plate. We can see cut ribs end on, with the intercostal muscles in between: two sets, crossing at right angles—the flesh familiar to eaters of beef or pork ribs. In breathing, one set raises the ribs, the other lowers them.

As the rib plate comes off, there is an eye-catching circular bruise on the tissues beneath, about two inches in diameter.

"Now what's that?" one student says. An instructor passing by stops and looks. He presses down on the bruise with the little-finger side of his gloved fist.

"Looks like CPR," he says, meaning the chest compressions for cardiopulmonary resuscitation. "I imagine someone tried to save this guy . . . and failed. What did he die of?"

"MI." Myocardial infarction: heart attack.

"Yes, that's probably it. Often smaller ribs are broken in the process, but this guy's built like a cathedral."

Standing over to the side, I meet a stranger.

I say hello.

He returns my greeting and adds mysteriously, "I'm just stopping by to see how everyone is getting along."

I wonder at this, since he isn't visiting any of the tables. When I look questioningly at him, he says with a smile:

"I'm the embalmer."

"Oh."

It dawns on me that by "everyone" he means the cadavers he has prepared.

"How, um, are they getting along?" I ask in what I hope is a conversational tone.

"They seem to be doing just fine," he says.

REMOVING THE HEART

· · ·

OW WILL STEVE and Jonathan do? I wonder. Today the Team Bs must give their first presentations. Some Team A members also show up to hear about the dissected chest. As I enter the lab Steve and Jonathan are standing alertly by Table 3 in their lab coats, with bare legs and running shoes below—but no socks. I look around the room and see six teams of nervous presenters. This is the first time for them to show what they have learned to a lab instructor, a Ph.D. in anatomy who presumably has it all down cold. I learn later this isn't exactly true, since researchers in anatomy and physiology specialize so highly that often they have to review areas of the anatomy in order to teach general anatomy, but the students, who don't know this, feel only trepidation. Furthermore, the lab instructor can ask embarrassing questions or find fault with the dissection. And the whole process is semipublic, with other students listening, some coming right up to the table to watch along with the instructor. With the strict ten-minute limitation, Steve and Jonathan will have to be well organized to explain the structures of the chest prescribed by the syllabus.

I wish the guys the best of luck: "About all set?"

"Boy, you bet. We worked on it last night and all the hour just before"—which was why they weren't at the lecture. "We're in good shape," Jonathan says.

"Look at this—a tag made of cinnamon-flavored dental floss," Steve announces, twirling the tan thread he's attached to a blood vessel in the cadaver. (This marker will stay in the cadaver until the end of the course; it and other evidence of the students' work become part of a long, slow process by which the students claim the bodies into their own world of experience. I later think of this as a kind of domestication.)

I say, "Knock 'em dead," too late realizing that these words might not be the best for the circumstances. I then go to a far wall, watching from a distance, without putting any more pressure on the men who are about to perform for the first time.

The instructor starts with Table 2 this time, saying that it would be good to rotate who begins. Team B at Table 1 is disappointed, since they wanted to be done and gone. Now they have at least an hour of waiting, as five other teams must precede them. I ask if I may look into their cadaver. They agree, and I peer in, finding a clean and neat dissection.

"Do you want to hear our presentation?" John and Larry ask me.

"Sure," I say, and they are off and running, perhaps for the dozenth time. They really have it down: the structure of the ribs, the path of the nerves, the flow of blood, and the structure of the lungs, all, of course, in the requisite terminology.

But "my guys" are about to start: the instructor is leaving Table 2 and passing to Table 3. Steve has actually shaved for the occasion and Jonathan's baseball cap almost looks clean. Is this a new cap? Or does it just look cleaner from a distance?

Jonathan speaks first, describing the ribs. As he talks, he holds up a tightly curved first rib, from his bone box. He next refers to the articulated skeleton hanging conveniently nearby, demonstrating the bony relationships. Steve follows next, showing structures inside the chest of the cadaver. Then Jonathan takes up again, holding up a lung and explaining it. Somewhere in the midst of all this Jonathan looks over at me and raises his eyebrows (the "eyebrow flash," in the anthropologist's phrase) to indicate, *Hey, wow, we're really doing it!*

The men finish up, and the instructor asks a few questions. Then they all go out into the hall to receive their grade in private. It's a 6, the highest mark.

As the instructor moves over to the Fatless Man and his two dissectors, other students congratulate Jonathan and Steve.

"Nice job, guys."

"Sounded great."

I ask them how they thought it went.

"Real good, man, no sweat," Steve says. They are elated. "I'm starting to get into this stuff, Steven!" Jonathan crows.

Two women arrive at this table, in their lab coats and shorts. Steve and Jonathan introduce me to Team C, Lisa Cerilli and Jocelyne Oriole. Lisa has long, taffy-colored hair, Jocelyne a friendly smile. They wear shorts and the standard white lab coat. If they are nervous, it isn't apparent to me. Other Team B members are still presenting to instructors, but Team C can start their work at the tables that have finished. Although clearly eager to leave the lab, Steve and Jonathan introduce Lisa and Jocelyne to the body lying faceup before them.

"She's a great cadaver; just keep her nice and wet so she doesn't dry out," Jonathan explains. "Use this bottle and refill it if you need to. When you're done, wet her down good, put the blanket back on, and spray her again. Then put the plastic over it all.

"Not bad for someone who could barely touch the corpse on the first day, huh?" he boasts. "Now I like to *squish right in!*" He and Steve laugh raucously. And depart.

Lisa and Jocelyne take over, slowly turning back the skin flaps and muscles to become familiar with this chest. It will be their job to remove the heart, to dissect it, and to create their ten-minute presentation. Still shrouded in tissue, the heart stands like a huge bulb in the middle of the thorax. Lisa on one side and Jocelyne on the other identify what they take to be the remains of the thymus gland (large in children but shriveled in adults) on top of that bulb and begin to scrape off fat. Soon they cut open the parietal (or outer) pericardium, a paper-thin but tough membrane surrounding the heart.

"What did that lecture say about fluid?" Lisa asks, scratching behind her ear.

"Oh yeah—the lady had blood between the two layers of the pericardium. They had to get it out," Jocelyne recalls. Too much fluid—from bleeding, for example—is dangerous, a condition known as "pericardial tamponade" that can be fatal: the heart is crushed within its own sack by blood it should be sending out into the body.

The room seems to have a particular intensity today, and I find the same is true in the three other rooms. Taking out the heart is no light matter. Some days the tension is dispelled through jokes about Frankenstein or Dracula, but today is quiet, focused.

Jocelyne says quietly, "I am *not* eating meat tonight."

"Me neither," replies Lisa. They seem to tune to each other's controlled repugnance.

Next, Lisa and Jocelyne cut away the visceral pericardium, the inner (or serous) layer immediately covering the heart. Suddenly we can see the aortic arch, bulging upward from the heart, an off-white tube like a good-sized garden hose. The carotid arteries spring upward from it to supply the brain—a heavy user of oxygen—then the aorta turns downward and pipes along the spine to supply the lower body through many arterial branches.

The women cut away fat and find, on this slow treasure hunt, the other vessels. Today, students go back and forth between the cadaver and other cadavers, asking each other what's what, how to cut so-and-so, and building a group consensus that they are all on the right track.

"It's just like organic chemistry," Lisa says. "They throw you in, and you have to make the best of it. Actually it's the best way to learn, even if it is slow."

Jocelyne agrees. "You know, I don't feel I know the other regions half as well as the ones I do myself." Probably all the students would agree. To see and feel a structure helps to set it in the mind. Several students insist that I experience this feel (part of Foucault's famous "gaze"); they seem to sense that to watch only is to miss much. The women invite me to put on a glove and stick my forefinger into this aged heart. This time, it's the right atrium, the first chamber where the vena cava dumps blood from the body. It feels thin for the job of contracting 100,000 times a day (70×60 minutes $\times$ 24 hours), some 3.8 billion times for the lifetime of this 101-year-old woman.

Lisa and Jocelyne are reserved—quiet and methodical. Each time I walk into the lab I ask myself, What qualities in these students would I like in physicians treating me? In Lisa, I see a certain doggedness, a resolve to get to the bottom of each anatomy assignment; I'd like such a doctor, one who would not quit until she had figured out what was wrong with me. From Jocelyne, I'd value the kindness and empathy I sense in her. Jonathan? Hearty good humor, so infectious it would put me at ease. Steve? An animal intensity that somehow affirms the necessity of health. Can we order such things in our doctors? Strictly speaking, no, but I prize such qualities so much that when I myself fill out the forms as a new patient, whether medical or dental, I write, *Patient is nervous and appreciates full explanations and statements of concern.*

At some tables, it's snip, snip, snip as the cutters work with obsessive care. "Let's be sure what we're doing before we cut anything major," I hear them saying. At other tables, there is more of a slasher mentality: "Here, let's just open this right up—we can identify things later." Both approaches seem to work, although the snippers take more time and do neater work. I wonder whether the teams that have two persons of the same temperament work best, or if it's possible that one slasher and one snipper would make the ideal combination. And in my doctor? If it's my body that he or she is cutting on, I think I'd vote for the snipper.

Across the room, John and Larry give the final Team B presentation of the day, making their corresponding Team C last to start the heart dissection. Luckily, their cadaver has almost no internal fat, so their job goes quickly. Also, they are true slashers and have their cadaver's heart out in less than an hour.

At another table, the team seems to stretch the job out interminably, finally calling for the instructor to give them a hand.

"Well, look," he says. "You're just about there." He pulls the heart up smartly, pushing tissues apart with his fingers. "All you need to do is this," he says, snipping the last pulmonary vein.

"And there you are." He lifts the heart out of the chest. Are the students disappointed at not making that last cut—or relieved that he did it?

At another table, a woman says, "Look at this junk we found in our heart." She shows me dark material on a paper towel. "Here's chunks of dried blood" (which normally pools and clots in the dead heart), "and here's some atheromas" (long strips of fatty matter that plug up the coronary arteries).

"French fries and pizza, I bet," she says with a laugh.

IS THIS T-5 OR WHAT?

• • •

LET'S GET THIS damn thing done and presented," I overhear a student growl as I walk into the lab. He, and all the members of Team C—Lisa and Jocelyne included—are the only ones who have not made their first presentation. Furthermore, it is suddenly the fourth week of the semester, and the first examination period will be in two weeks. Since this exam will cover anatomy, physiology, and biochemistry, there's a lot to learn. Biochemistry is gaining favor as a scapegoat. The students find it abstract, esoteric—certainly compared with the hands-on nature of human anatomy—and, as only students can, they formulate comments of disgust and loathing about it.

Steve and Jonathan visit Lisa and Jocelyne, giving them tips for the presentation and picking up knowledge about the chest cavity and heart. Some of this information comes together by trial and error as students make formulations, correct them, and reach better formulations. The heavy cutting for this dissection is done; now it's a matter of refinement, poking with a probe, picking among the fine structures. At the six tables in Room 1, work typically divides like this: one student trims away at the removed heart while the other tidies up the cavern of the chest. Students compare structures to their texts or to other cadavers nearby.

As they peer into the chest someone asks, "How do we know what's what in here? Is this T-5 or what?" The twelve thoracic vertebrae (one per rib)

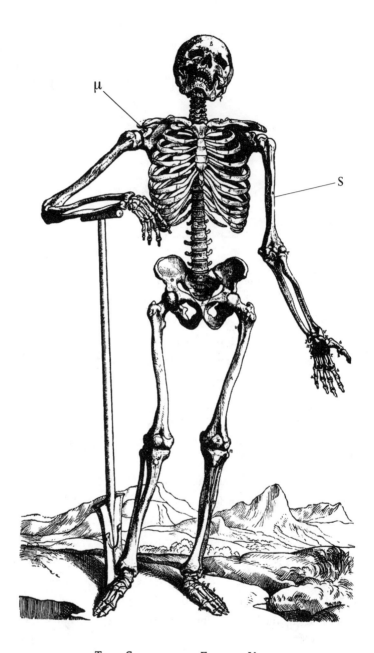

μ

S

THE SKELETON: FRONT VIEW

(Figure 10)

From *De fabrica*, page 163.

LIKE THE MUSCLEMEN, the skeleton stands on his own and in a landscape. He has, however, a prop with him, a shovel suitable (despite the crooked handle) for digging graves. Saunders and O'Malley perceive an open grave here as well and attribute the figure of the *danse macabre* or Death itself to all these signs (page 84).

Furthermore, while acknowledging the basic success of the illustration, they see errors in proportion, such as a too-short torso and too-long arms.

The skeleton is a male (see the sharp upward V at the base of the pelvis) seventeen or eighteen years old.

The coracoid ("crow-shaped") prominence of the scapula (shoulder blade) is marked with the Greek letter mu ("μ") near the left shoulder, where the upper arm bone (humerus—marked "S") joins.

At birth, a human has some 350 bones. Many of these eventually fuse, yielding, on average, 206 to 208 in an adult.

obviously don't come numbered; because they slant downward as they come around from the back, they are confusing without the rib plate in place.

Jocelyne shows Steve and Jonathan the mediastinal (central chest) cavity, the nerves, the blood vessels, and the thoracic duct, which brings the clear fluid lymph from much of the body back to the heart to be mixed back into the circulating blood. Steve and Jonathan offer what they know from their initial dissection, and slowly the students build up their understanding of the body, as carefully as they have torn down the physical structures.

Lisa holds up the heart for the two men.

"Okay, let's get oriented here," she says. "This is anterior wall, and this is aorta, up here, and here right below is left atrium, and left ventricle below that, with nice thick walls. Right ventricle is next to it, and right atrium above." She turns the heart one way and another, as if working a Rubik's Cube, except that the heart is more egg-shaped than cubic, and the parts stay in place. Such is the ritual for examination of the heart, even the phrase "getting oriented." The heart, especially when partially covered with fat, is confusing to look at—a big, globby fist—with nothing like the clarity of, say, a human head. It certainly bears no resemblance to the traditional valentine heart! So students and anatomy instructors alike will take a heart in hand and intone, "Let's get oriented," often starting at the aorta, the largest vessel springing from what must be the top.

Jonathan asks, "So if this heart were in your body, how would it be?" Lisa holds the heart in front of her chest, pointing the apex (the conical end) down and then slightly to the left. The orientation is not only to "what is what" in the heart, but also to "what is where." Lisa holds the heart, cold, still, and isolated, a scant three inches from her own heart, warm, pulsing, and hooked within her body by nerves and the eight major vessels. Indeed, students point to their own bodies more and more; they say things like "It runs across here, and up" and trace the path on their white coats. Thus orientation is not only to direction (some absolute "sunrise," in the original sense of "orient"), but to a web of interconnections within the cadaver and, increasingly, between corpse and living person. The students complain that biochemistry is abstract; by contrast, anatomy is immediate and tactile. Lisa waves her hand in the cadaver's chest and says, "With this stuff, you get to play with it."

When Lisa talks about physical structures she often omits an article, according to common medical usage. Thus she says "right ventricle," not "the right ventricle." The poetic term for this is "ellipsis," and its effect is a sense of universality, as if to look at one aorta is to look at all of them, dead or alive, in this room or around the world, on this day in September or throughout all human time.

But, as I see progress, the Team C members feel their confidence at a low ebb. Teams A and B have already presented, that is to say, *everyone* has presented except for them. Many of the Team Cs feel the frustration of trying to learn everything in order to present it on Thursday, certainly too much, too quickly! They may sound knowledgeable as they present informally to their peers, but they feel insecure. "I'm so sick of this heart," one moans. "I've spent so much time on it and it's still confusing. Why didn't we get something easy, like the back?"

"Okay," Lisa continues, "if you look in here, you can see tricuspid valves."

"Oh, my God. That's so neat!" Jonathan bursts out. "That's them, just like the drawings. Boy, they're big. And this is a hundred-and-one-year-old heart. Can you imagine? It beat for over a century!" (I thought Jonathan and Steve had dashed out of here, but instead they have been touring the heart exhibits in the other rooms for an hour.) They are examining the valves through the slits Lisa and Jocelyne made the previous evening. Here's the mitral valve, so named because it resembles a bishop's miter, a conical cap. Here are the two semilunar valves, which release blood to the pulmonary arteries. All four valves open and close in response to a complex dance of electricity that runs through the heart; working in pairs, they make noise as they open and close. Physicians discern four normal heart sounds, of which the first two are the most well known—often styled as *lub dub.* (Artificial valves, made of a ball within rings and wires, give clicking sounds, and show up in X rays as dramatic bright white because of their opacity.) That night I use a stethoscope to listen to my own heart. I hear the bass drum *lub*, and then the higher, more precise pitch, *dub*, more like a kettle drum. It sounds like a waltz, with an absent third beat: *boom, bam, rest, boom, bam, rest*—the constant triple rhythm that keeps us alive, as the valves and walls pulse at various tempos—fast waltz, slow waltz—day and night.

If the first day on the heart was intense and physical, this second day is focused and verbal. I stand at the edge of the room and watch twenty-three students clustered around six tables, chattering away, hearts and probes in hand. They are bringing language together with the structures before them. I close my eyes and hear an anatomical babble, not the noise of the unfinished Tower of Babel, but the inspiring sound of constructive inquiry. This is what education should be: student-centered, experiential, cooperative, additive, with built-in rewards. As an outsider, I am envious.

The only figure in the room at all parallel to me seems to be Mr. Bones, the articulated skeleton at the far end of the aisle, hanging from the chain at the top of his skull. (It is a "he," I've discovered, looking at the upward V notch of his pelvis, not the gentle female U; see Figure 10 above.) But no, even he is more involved, as two students settle an argument about ribs and vertebrae, tracing his bones with their fingers. I too have touched him today, trying to verify the claim of the anatomy book that the coracoid prominence of the scapula (shoulder blade) may be felt from the front of the body. What a ridiculous claim, I thought, since the scapula is clearly on the back. Indeed, I have made the hollow of my upper chest sore, poking just under the clavicle (collarbone) out toward the head of the humerus (the upper arm bone). As I look at the skeleton, suddenly it is all magically clear: the coracoid ("crow-shaped") prominence pokes forward like the beak of a bird; I touch my chest through my shirt, more gently this time, and feel the thing. Bone, word, and touch all coalesce to insight.

It turns out that beside the sink is a good place for me to stand, since a parade of hearts comes to be washed.

"How's your heart?" I ask the students, acutely aware of the ambiguity of "your." They hold up the cadaveric hearts immediately, patting them gently with paper towels, eager to show off features they now understand.

"Well, ours is pretty small, which made dissection difficult, but here's . . ."

And: "This guy did *not* follow good health habits, I would say. He cost us a lot of time in getting the fat off of his heart."

And: "Look at this: here's his heart attack." Jenifer shows me a coronary artery that wiggles along the top of the heart, then suddenly stops. Below it the color and texture of the heart muscle are different: darker, slacker. Something blocked that artery, perhaps an embolus or a dissecting atheroma.

"See, the tissue below all died without oxygen. Killed him." I feel a wave of emotion: we have just seen this man's final fatal secret.

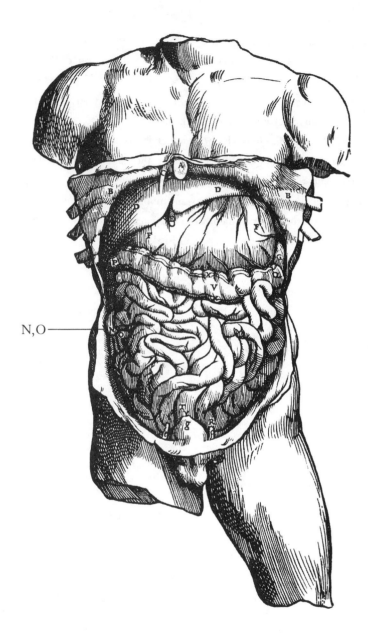

N,O

THE OPENED ABDOMEN

(Figure 11)

From *De fabrica*, page 360.

In its outlines, the figure is reminiscent of a fragment of Greek sculpture, but the opened abdomen has a dramatic novelty unknown in classical art. Here, the ribs are pulled back and the omentum (the fatty, overlying apron) is removed. The liver ("D") stretches across the top, with its falciform ligament ("E"). The stomach (rather enormous) is marked by "F," and the spleen, to its right, by "G." Just below is the transverse colon ("V"), and then the small intestine. Letters "N" and "O" indicate the caecum, or "blind" joining of the small and large bowels and (hard to make out) the appendix. The letter "g" indicates the urinary bladder.

A modern anatomist viewing this engraving suggested that the remarkable size of the stomach could be due to gases of decomposition in the cadaver.

THE TRIUMPHANT RETURN
OF TEAM A
• • •

W E GOT A real tough one, a real bitch," a student says to me as we walk up the stairs. His cadaver died of cancer, some of which, he thinks, has left fibrous material around the heart. He adds, "Our presentation is only forty seconds over. We're hoping the instructor won't notice."

In the anatomy lab, the teams have typically divided their presentations the same way they divided the cutting chores, between the chest specialists and the heart specialists. They are practicing their presentations to the other members of the teams. Although the room is full of students, it doesn't seem crowded, since each table has two talkers and four intent listeners, all closely clustered around the cadaver.

"I just love this," Kathy says at Nero's table. "You can just swoop in and gain the benefit of hours of work by the other guys. And you really appreciate it, knowing what it takes to get it all together!"

Steve and Jonathan are at Table 3, listening to Jocelyne and Lisa. Cliff Grossman and David Carlton, Team A, the two men who originally did the back dissection on Little Old Lady, are there also. As she speaks, Jocelyne points into the chest cavity with a probe; Lisa turns the heart in her hands, opening the various slits to show the chambers and valves. Suddenly the instructor enters the lab and heads toward Lisa and Jocelyne. Table 3 is first up today. I leave them, heading to a far corner.

At Table 1, Dave and Chris have worked a .22-caliber bullet into their routine, which they are giving to their teammates and anyone else who will listen: "This lady presented at the emergency room at one A.M. last night in severe pain. . . ." Their story includes the removal of this bullet from the pericardial walls by emergency surgery.

"We thought it would be good to introduce a little drama into our presentation," they say. "The instructor is likely to be worn down by hearing four versions of the heart before getting to us. Gotta spice things up."

The bullet does indeed lend a certain drama, even with its shiny casing that indicates it has never been fired. When they are finished with their ten-minute presentation I remark how clean their dissection looks.

"Well, we really lucked out. This is a great body. She got an experimental embalming treatment, and she's holding up great." (I learn later that the balance of chemicals was changed for her.) Their modesty aside, they have obviously used great care: the fat is meticulously removed, and the inside of the chest is neatly prepared. I look across the room and find Lisa and Jocelyne still presenting to the instructor, ten, twelve, fourteen minutes now going by. Finally, after sixteen minutes, the instructor stands up. They all go out into the hall for evaluation. The women return elated: their score is a 6. Their classmates congratulate them.

"I'm going shopping!" Lisa announces.

I stop by Nero's table, where Brad and Alex are chatting. "How's it going; all set to present?"

"Yeah, I think so. Want to hear it?"

"Sure."

So they begin alternating between the chest and the heart. They are terrific. As Alex turns the heart to show me the inner workings, another student enters the lab and greets me. When I attempt to sneak a "Hi" over Alex's shoulder, he pivots his eyes from the heart to my face, as if to ask, *Hey, are you really in this?*

"Right, right," I assure him (and myself), "the mitral valve. Right." Alex continues with his presentation. Near the end, he pulls back his lab coat (Clark Kent style) to reveal a T-shirt on which he has drawn the ribs and heart, with indications of heart sounds in red and the valves in green. Brad thumps the various areas to explain how it all works. Surely this team will do fine. I feel focus and intensity in their work. I would want my physician to be like these young people, really involved in whatever concern I would bring to him or her. It's only recently, in fact, that my physician has been younger than I am. My regular doc, wonderful Dr. Pryor, suddenly died of a heart attack, stunning all of us. I realized that I had made him a symbolic barrier against death, and when he was precipitously gone, I felt unprotected. My next doc, whom I now admire and trust, seemed at first like a kid. How could he protect me from death? Would his youth be pushing me ahead of him to my demise? I look at these students around the room and try to imagine myself telling them of chest pains, a swollen joint, a racking cough. Would they know what to do?

The presentations finish up around the room. The students who have presented on other days are generous in their praise, with claps on the back, even hugs. Team C is jelling as a social entity of twelve people working together in this room.

"Way to go."

"Super clear."

"Nice job."

Compared to the first presentations on the back, these on the heart and chest are crisper and more imaginative. Evidently the students are feeling more at home in this strange room.

But not every presentation is a success. At one table the students receive a 5, and they are stunned. I can't imagine that one single point would make any difference in their final grade: the tragedy must be, in their eyes, symbolic. Perhaps one clue is that both men have worn dress shirts and ties under their lab coats—professional garb. After so much work, strategy, and a competent ten-minute performance, they are, somehow, "second-rate." Other students come and say, "Shake it off," "You know the stuff," "It doesn't really make any difference," but this team is disconsolate and leaves glumly.

Cliff and David take over Table 3. The first to return to work in the lab, they seem comfortable with text, tools, and cadaver: Team A returns in triumph. They get right to work on the abdomen, a volume often treacherous because of its stores of fat. Consulting their carefully marked texts, they start to peel back the skin on their cadaver's belly to trim out the fat. I ask them how it was turning over the body on the very first day.

"It was bad, man, so totally different. I didn't want to touch her," Cliff exclaims. He's an intense man with glasses and brown hair. But now both men are touching and cutting as if they did this every day.

"Was this the body of a hundred-and-one-year-old?" a student from another room asks. This cadaver, the oldest of all the cadavers, has gained some notoriety. "Yes . . . and still is," David says, matter-of-factly. We all chuckle, perhaps wondering whether this is still *her* body.

David says, "You know, I asked the instructor about her age. I thought that a hundred-and-one-year-old cadaver would be bad news . . . all falling apart and hard to work on, but he said, 'Just the opposite—anyone that old would probably be a good specimen, just by being healthy that long.' "

There are more jokes today than ever before. At one table a veteran chides a tentative cutter: "You hold the tools like you're eating dinner!" I stop at a neighboring table where the laughter is dying down and ask what I missed. As an outsider, I am not likely to be in on the jokes, but I wheedle until I learn that the joke is about the male cadaver's genitals and, given their size, whether his brains were positioned there also. "Old crotch-brains, huh? How *unusual*," I venture.

"That's him. And not at all unusual." We laugh. The repartee continues, moving into the realm of stories of "borrowed" parts from medical labs. One story involves a tollbooth, where a collector received quarters. Some wise-guy med students, the story runs, took the hand and arm from a cadaver and presented their toll with it, to the horror of the collector. This time no one laughs full out; people just shake their heads, uttering small *heh-hehs*. Another student mentions the case of an entire head taken from an anatomy lab. This brought down an investigation by "a large number of police agencies," he says gravely. Even if such anecdotes are merely urban legend, they seem to reflect accurately our culture's nervousness about dead bodies.

Now that the students are working their way down the body to the pelvis and perineum, they can no longer ignore the sexuality of their cadavers. For the back and even the chest (female breasts were turned back with the wings of the skin), the cadavers had no sexual identity, with the possible exception of Nero, who seems so powerful that it is hard to forget his sex. The Neronian cutters suggest delicately that he must have been "a real ladies' man." "Or a baseball player," someone jokes. "Yeah, well, I bet he hit home runs," another replies.

After the initial incisions in the belly and the peeling back of the skin, the Team A members find it's slow going today, especially trying to discriminate the layers of fascia that cover the thin stomach muscles. The muscles taper away, becoming a single tough, translucent membrane.

"Remove all remains of the superficial fascia," Cliff reads from the *Dissector*. "Easy for them to say," he mutters, clipping away. Somehow it always sounds plausible and reasonable in the book. The complexities of a particular corpse, however, are myriad, with layers grown together, individual oddities, vague landmarks, scar tissue, and results of disease processes.

Cliff and David invite me to put on a glove to feel some of the structures, and I remember to glove my left hand this time, so I can still take notes with my right. I like being more involved. Sometimes I look things up in the anatomy books for the students, who don't want to smear "cadaver juice" on their expensive books. I adjust a lamp. Sometimes Cliff asks me to take his glasses off his face before they fall into the open torso of his cadaver.

Eventually Cliff and David have trimmed down to the external obliques, have cleaned off the two central bands of muscle (the rectus abdominis) running vertically from the ribs to the pubis, and have located the inguinal canal. "Must be the round ligament in here," Cliff says, showing this canal slanting across the lower abdomen. (In a male, it would be the spermatic cord on its curving journey up from the testes into the pelvis; the round ligament helps support the uterus, so called to distinguish it from the broad ligament, which shares in the same function.)

I wander around and find other groups cutting away with parallel problems in the abdominal coverings, all except for the Outpost, the nineteenth table in a room by itself. Joan is tapping her probe on her corpse, whose musculature is *all* pulled back. *Wow*—there's the liver, the stomach, and lots of intestines, all bulging out of the abdominal cavity. (See Figure 11 above.)

"Can you help me with this?" she asks, raising her dark eyebrows.

"I wish I could," I say and give my little speech about merely observing. "But I don't mind looking with you, if it's okay." We poke around in the guts and make some reasonable guesses. It sure seems crowded in there. What would it be like with food as well? Perhaps the embalming bloats things up? Certainly the muscle layers once held things more in place.

"My dad's a surgeon, and he repairs hernias," Joan says. "I've got a lot more respect for what he does now, seeing how complicated this all is. For a direct hernia—were you in the lecture?" I say yes.

"Right. Well, the direct hernia would go through here, and the indirect would go like this," she shows the muscle layers. Her teammate returns from her futile trip in the other rooms to see how other teams are handling their viscera, but no other teams have gotten this far. (*Viscera* is the fancy word for hollow organs, straight from the Latin: properly, several *viscera*, but one *viscus*.) Before long an anatomy instructor, Dr. John McDonald, stops by and leads both students through identification of organs, structures, and openings. He is careful not to do the work for them ("And this is this and that is that") but does it heuristically: "And if this is this, what would that *have* to be?" so that the students make the discoveries for themselves.

The stomach is a slack pouch, surprisingly mobile, but the large intestine is stuck to tissues below by adhesions. McDonald pulls it free with his gloved hand. The liver seems very large—perhaps diseased—and green bile has leaked below it, staining the tissues there. The entire digestive area seems to have its own genius: organs fitting into each other in a three-dimensional choreography. The cadaveric guts are stilled now, of course, but our guts move in us, the four living persons around the table. Our lunch is mostly in our stomachs now, but breakfast is churning along our bowels through peristaltic action, as the sections of bowel signal ahead by nerve and enzyme that more food is coming.

It may all seem very slow, but the Team As are cutting away with a vigor much different from the tremulous first day. Nineteen abdomens are opened quickly, and many of the teams feel free to stop at five o'clock, since they can finish off later "with no sweat," as Cliff says. He and David wet their cadaver down and cover her up and depart.

IT'S SO GREAT TO
SEE ALL THIS STUFF!

• • •

HE LECTURE TODAY was about the vasculature of the abdomen, and the guest lecturer certainly knew his stuff. His slides showed new techniques for X-raying blood vessels and for treatments of blood-vessel disease. Since the arteries and veins have roughly the same density as organs, they don't show up on X ray unless there is a "contrast material" injected into them. The lecturer showed a picture of the slender catheters through which an iodine solution could be precisely released into a vessel. Like the calcium of bones, the iodine is more dense than the usual carbon, hydrogen, and nitrogen of soft tissue; therefore it absorbs more X rays, making an artery and its distribution appear a dramatic white on film, snaking and branching, like an aerial photo of the Mississippi Delta.

Regrettably, however, our guest was not an exhilarating speaker. Indeed the lecture hall, darkened more than usual for his particular slides, seemed a fine prospect for a siesta. But the students were alert, and the questions, raised during his talk and after, were precise. At the end of the talk the students applauded. The lecturer even commented that this was unusual. *What's happening?* I wondered. Perhaps the best answer was that the students were a few more steps along the medical road. They have not yet dissected down to the descending aorta and its arterial branches, but now they'll know what to look for when they get there. Knowing that some of their cadavers died of various kinds of vascular disease (*vascular* comes from the Latin for "small

(Figure 12)

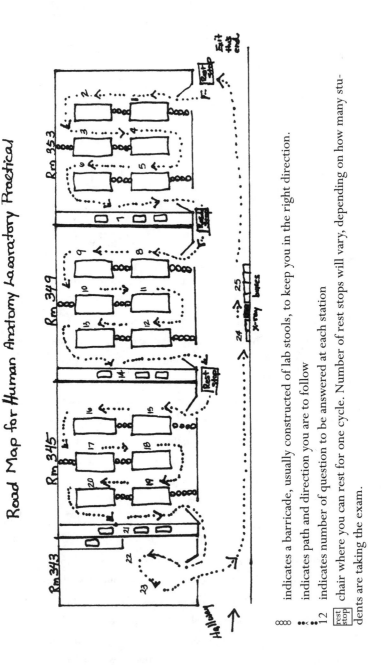

indicates a barricade, usually constructed of lab stools, to keep you in the right direction.

indicates path and direction you are to follow

12 indicates number of question to be answered at each station

rest stop chair where you can rest for one cycle. Number of rest stops will vary, depending on how many students are taking the exam.

(Diagram by Barbara Brown, Ph.D., Human Anatomy Course Syllabus, 1989, Emory University, page 27. Used by permission.)

vessel," here for blood), they pay attention when the lecturer, even with his flat, midwestern voice, tells them about the illnesses his techniques can diagnose.

The black-and-white slides flash by, showing elaborate patterns of white lines that branch and fan, like trees without leaves. Vascular radiography can show aneurysms (arterial bulges), occlusions (blockages), and tumors (growths revealed by vessels being pushed aside). Several of these conditions can be treated right away through the same catheter; for example, a drug may be injected at the site of a bleeding artery to make it close up, or a narrow balloon inflated to block off a vein that has lost its valves. This fine plumbing can save a patient a major abdominal operation and days or even weeks in the hospital.

Up in the lab, it's another "talking" day. The major aims of this dissection have been met over the weekend. Cliff and David, for example, have done a lot of cutting, and their cadaver is "in good shape," as they say, an ironic phrase for a body about to be disemboweled. Jonathan and Steve are there, in remarkably high spirits, and Lisa too. There's a little horseplay in the hall, as Jonathan puts a friendly choker grip around Lisa's neck. Everyone seems in a good mood, despite the impending exams for the first third of the course.

These will constitute the "Joint Examination" on Monday morning, followed by an anatomy lab exam that afternoon. There are predictable jokes about the "joint" exam—that it will concern the knee joint, or that everyone will smoke marijuana—but it represents an ideal the faculty have, to ask questions that combine the three main courses, anatomy, physiology, and biochemistry. The students seem to have no idea whether such a synthesis is possible: they are scrambling to learn the basics for each of the courses separately. Today, then, there is a strong practical interest in learning all the body structures, and most of the team members, once again, are clustered around the tables, where Team A holds forth, showing what they have learned. Groups also make plans to meet to study. Whose apartment? What time?

Cliff and David flank the table, and Cliff does most of the talking. Their dissection is careful and clear. This cadaver even smells right, since it is now, for me, the norm. Some of the other corpses smell bad to me, but not this one. Some of the visitors from other tables, however, wrinkle their noses and complain.

Cliff explains the muscle layers on the front of the abdomen, where they begin and end, how they are innervated, and their blood supply. He turns these back and shows the inguinal tunnel and the landmarks of the viscera underneath. All this takes a long time, as the students add points, raise questions, even disagree; typically they turn to anatomy texts to "get this settled." Furthermore, there are more students from other rooms than ever before, so Cliff keeps doing his routine for different audiences. He explains, and explains—for one hour and fifteen minutes.

The other tables are similar. The Team A members who did the dissection explain the structures for their classmates—and for anyone else who is looking in. At the next table, a student listens to the story of Nero's immense abdomen so intently that he seems unaware that his hand leans directly on the blanket overlying Nero's face.

At the table on the other side, Stephen Lee says, "It's so great to see all this stuff after reading about it for years!" He puts his gloved hand into the viscera, pokes, and identifies the elements of the g-i (gastro-intestinal) tract and associated organs. There's the stomach, an empty bag; there on the cadaver's left is the liver, huge, appearing much like a calf's liver in the supermarket; and there on the other side is the spleen, a small purple sac, much smaller than when active in life. In the Middle Ages, the spleen was considered the source of black bile or melancholy. Lying under *(hypo)* the rib cartilages *(chondros),* it has been considered the source of undue concern about health, or *hypochondria.*

Hiding in the lobes of the liver is the gallbladder; most of these are bright green from leaking bile. Way down in the middle is a glimpse of a pink finger, the pancreas. Stephen and his colleagues follow the large bowel down to the connection with the small bowel: the appendix should be here, if it hasn't shriveled or been removed.

"Is that it?" someone asks, pointing to a thin, wormlike (vermiform) tube.

"You betcha," another replies.

Back at Table 3, Cliff and David invite me to "take a feel." I put on a glove and grope around.

"Try the pyloric sphincter," they say. "It's really neat." I feel the lower valve of the stomach, finding it a resilient ring. When it works right, this structure keeps the dilute hydrochloric acid within the stomach, faithfully releasing only small amounts of food into the duodenum to begin their long voyage through the bowels. When this valve doesn't work right, it can release sufficient acid to nourish the bacteria that cause a duodenal ulcer.

At the next table, Mei looks with her dark eyes from her guts to ours. "I just love the g-i tract," she says, flashing her wide smile.

This dissection calls for pulling one of the testes from the scrotum up into the abdomen to dissect its major structures. This certainly sounds odd, but it makes anatomical sense because, in the embryo, the testes descend from an area near the kidneys, taking abdominal layers with them. Surgery on the testes often starts with an incision in the lower abdomen. From Table 3, Steve, Jonathan, and I look over at another table, where a woman holds a testicle in her hand and pokes at it with her probe.

"Don't you *hate* it when they squeeze the testicle like that?" Jonathan whispers and several of us males make faces and shudder in agreement. In the female cadavers, there is the goal of finding the round ligament going through the inguinal canal; it seems to be a fine structure, hard to be sure of. At one table, the students ask an instructor, Dr. Jim Wilson, "Can we borrow you for a moment?"

"Sure. What do you need?"

"Is this the round ligament? I'm not even sure if this is the inguinal canal or whether I just created it," Pete says, pointing with his probe to the surface of the lower abdomen. Pete is an exceptionally tall man—his nickname is Condor. When he sits on the stool to dissect, his upper body hunches over the cadaver to bring his intent face near.

"Well, it might be," Wilson replies, "but I always approach the round ligament from the parietal well." He puts his gloved hands inside the lower abdomen of the corpse and starts to pull the intestines around.

"A few adhesions," he mutters, pulling the intestines from the abdominal wall and from each other, leaving their snaky structures intact. A quiet man, he is tall and, it seems, strong, since the cadaver moves and the stainless-steel table shakes. I hear tearing sounds.

"There, now we have room to see what we're doing."

He pulls back the outer tissue and shows, from below, where the round ligament should be. With a few pokes of a probe, he isolates a string the size of yarn. "I think that's it." There are a few more interchanges, and he departs.

"Doesn't that piss you off," Pete says to Bill. "The instructor knows all the neat shortcuts the books say nothing about. We could have spent hours snipping our way into that!"

I visit all the corpses in the room. At one table I meet a strawberry-blond woman with bright blue eyes.

"I'm going to see *all* the bodies today!" she announces. I ask her whether there's much difference. "Oh yes, stuff's in different places; and we'll need to know that when it comes to the lab exam, since we'll be looking into all the cadavers."

She's right. The syllabus shows a floor plan leading students through all the tables, where various structures will be labeled for identification (see Figure 12 above).

She looks into one open abdomen. "Oh, your liver is a different color from ours. This looks like what you get at the store, you know, to cook. And you can see your caudate [the taillike part of the liver] really well."

I too wander through the other rooms. Here's an immensely fat cadaver, with gobbets of fat hanging from every internal fold. Here's a cadaver missing a spleen. This one has half of the large bowel gone, removed by surgery. That cadaver is shot through with cancerous growths. There are so many ways to die, it appears, but we don't seem to have any traumatic deaths, as in automobile wrecks. I have seen internal medicine texts three inches thick that give in hundreds of pages the infinite number of things that can go wrong with our bodies; they are dreary reading. And still, all these cadavers, from whatever cause, are equally dead. All of them, regardless of their position in life, despite their "net worth" (a phrase I despise), despite any desires they might have had to keep on living or, conversely, to die—all have left mortal remains that are equally dead, but wonderfully different in what they now display. These differences are in part mysterious, in part explainable through the anatomical variations that they were born with, that developed during their long lives, or that developed as these bodies began to leave the world of the living for the world of the dead.

TO SPRITZ ALL BODIES

• • •

ODAY IS VERY different from any previous day, for this is Review Day, and it signals the impending written and practical exams. The time of pure, unaccountable learning is drawing to an end, and the general anxiety level is rising. The students are aware of this and use me as a measure: "You don't have to take the exam, do you?" Their nervous jokes are also on the increase.

Today's meeting is even physically different. We are in a smaller lecture room, sitting closer together than usual to each other and to the instructor, Art English, our leader for the review. No other instructors are there, and I sit with Jonathan, Steve, Mei, Cliff, and Allison. Everyone is anxious and attentive, since today the rules for the exam are to be made clear. I have heard many complain: "There's just too much to learn." Others have said, "It comes so fast, you don't even have time to think what it means." Because Pedagogy of Overload is standard for graduate schools in general, and for medicine in particular, the end result, as everyone knows, is Pervasive Stress.

"If you've been keeping up, you should have no trouble," English tells the apprehensive students. "All of the questions will be from the objectives listed for Dissection One through Four. When we meet as a faculty to make up this exam, each professor proposing a question *must* tell which objective it involves." English also explains the mechanics of the exam, with four groups of students (alphabetically created) rotating through the lab. There are to be twenty-five stations, typically exhibits in cadavers (but also some X rays along the side of the room) with tags to mark something—a bone, a nerve, a muscle, a blood vessel—and five choices to choose from for each exam question.

"As Dr. Wolf noted when we went to this system, we always provide you with the right answers. Furthermore, you don't have to worry about your spelling or handwriting. The spelling will come and the handwriting we can't do anything about anyway," he quips.

"Now let's review a little building anatomy," English says, and someone laughs. "I'll remember your face," English jokes, pointing to the student.

"Do we need pencils or pens?" a student interrupts.

"No, they will be supplied."

"Ohhh!" the students respond in mock gratitude.

"You must be getting something for all this tuition," says English.

Place aux jeunes, the students are saying, or *Move over, old man,* as well as *We're nervous about all this.* English is conveying something like: *I'll joke with you to recognize your nervousness and assure you that we are trying to make this test fair and efficient.*

"As you come up the elevators on the anatomy side of the building," he continues, "there will be someone to greet you and lead you to your station area."

"A kind of tour guide?" a student calls out.

"Well, yes. It's all part of being a modern scientist," English banters back.

"Should we already have on our lab coats as we get off the elevator?" Loud cheers from the students at this insight into the elaborate process!

"Yes . . . and all of you remember *his* name," English splices to the earlier joke.

The students are to take the forty-minute exam and "then descend down the physiology side, so that the euphoric and the anxious groups don't meet: it's best to keep these two populations apart," English says. His phrase is so well turned that I wonder how many see through it: to keep apart those who have seen the test from those who are about to take it, clearly a point where cheating might be possible.

"Will someone spritz our bodies to keep them from drying out?" It's hard to tell whether this is a completely ingenuous question or, more likely, another challenging barb. Certainly the bodies will be open and drying for the three hours of the exam, but this is no longer than any of the labs have been so far.

"Yes, among our many duties during the afternoon, we will spritz all bodies," English replies. English is referring to the nineteen cadavers, of course, but given the ambiguity of which bodies we're talking about, I wonder about a symbolic spritzing of all 113 students, a sprinkling of pedagogical juice during this review hour that will help them on the exam.

"Will yesterday's lecture be on it?"

"Only if it relates to the Learning Objectives for Dissections One through Four. Yesterday's lecture was on the deep vasculature of the abdomen. Those structures are not in these objectives, therefore, that lecture will not be on the exam. That's the kind of reasoning you should use. If you put your minds to it, you can probably guess much of the exam."

"How are we going through all the stations at once?"

"Okay, how many of you have taken a cafeteria-style or stationed exam before?" English asks.

About 75 percent of the hands go up.

"Well, maybe I should ask how many of you have not?"

The remainder of hands go up.

"The first group can take a nap while I talk to the second. You will spread out over twenty-five stations at the start. Let's say you start on Thirteen; obviously you will want to start your answer sheet with Thirteen. At the sound of a bell, or sedate tone—what do we have this year?" he wonders out loud.

"Electroshock?" a student yells. The room rings with laughter.

"Oh yes, we just got that working again this year—all the tables are wired."

"Will the stations be numbered?" Many students turn around to stare at this man, who blushes hotly. There is nervous laughter.

"Yes. They are definitely numbered," English replies, not joking back.

There are some more details, but the questions fizzle out after nineteen minutes into the hour and English proceeds to give a practice examination. The lights dim and pairs of slides come on; on the large screens in front of us we find on the left a color photo of an anatomical exhibit with a single structure indicated by a line and a number; on the right is a slide of a typed page, a multiple-choice question with five answers. The first one, a transverse section of a heart, has a valve tagged. The accompanying question reads like this:

> The tagged structure in the heart is:
> A. The posterior mitral valve
> B. The anterior mitral valve
> C. The medial leaflet of the tricuspid valve
> D. The posterior leaflet of the tricuspid valve
> E. The anterior leaflet of the tricuspid valve

Suddenly it's very quiet in the room. All eyes are riveted to the front, and I can see heads swiveling back and forth between the two screens. *What must they be thinking,* I wonder, and start my own guessing. The top of the heart shows the aortic arch bending away ("Let's get oriented here"), so we must be viewing the heart upright and from the front. That would make the lower chamber the *right* (always from the patient's or cadaver's point of view) ventricle—which is verified by the thinner cardiac walls (it pumps to the lungs, not the whole body). The valve must be the tricuspid, then. Since we can only see the front leaflet, it must be the anterior leaflet. I write down "E," imagining that the students have followed a similar line of reasoning, only much more quickly.

The pairs of slides continue, with a coronary artery, a branch of the vagus nerve, various other nerves, intercostal muscles, an "impression" on a lung, a ligament between the liver and stomach, then the falciform ("sickle-shaped") ligament of the liver.

"Ahhhhhh," the collective group breathes in gratitude, since that's an easy one. Then some fascia in the lower abdomen, muscles along the spine, another nerve, and three questions about vertebrae. Many of the questions are more than simple identifications, since there are combinations of A and C, or B and C, even combining types of knowledge. For example, a nerve needs the correct name as well as information about its neurotransmitter. After the sixteenth slide, English breaks in.

"Okay, now let's go through these again, and I'll share something of my personal philosophy on how to take an exam like this," he says. "First, the actual exhibits will be easier, since you will have the entire cadaver right there, with no vignetting, as in these slides. The slides clearly restrict our vision, limiting perception of scale and context. With a cadaver, you can change your angle of vision; you can't see depth in these slides. This is a case in which the real is easier." I think of Foucault's famous "gaze," but that was largely influenced by technological changes such as the stethoscope and X rays; by contrast, the anatomy lab is low-tech, with direct sight, smell, and touch.

English then marches through the slides, modeling a reasoning process for identification, elimination of false answers, and verification of the best hypotheses. Occasional questions from the students challenge his answer, presumably from the students who got it wrong, and English clarifies why the right answer is right, why the wrong won't do. In sum, English is serving as a tutor to the entire class, bringing them toward peak form for Monday. As the discussion of the last slides on the vertebrae finishes up, English urges the students, "Get close to your bone box."

The job is done; the class is over early, since no one has any more questions.

"How does it look?" I ask a student.

"Hey, we're on top of it. Anatomy makes sense: you put the words together with the objects. It's that goddamn biochem we can't hack."

WITH LONG HAIR DOWN

· · ·

XAMINATION DAY. THE students have studied during the weekend, in groups or alone. Some have done little else, while others may have calculated the appropriate minimal effort. There is anxiety, but there is also momentum; after all, these are sharp and highly motivated people. They have done well in hundreds of tests before, and their futures as physicians depend on passing tests like these both here in med school and in various certifying and recertifying exams in the future. I imagine there are some who are behind in their work, but they are not obvious to me. I make no effort to visit the morning exam, which I picture as the usual dreary marking of computer forms.

The laboratory exam seems promising, however, so I drop by in the afternoon. The students arrive in the four alphabetically prescribed groups, forty minutes apart. They have on their white coats, but, underneath, most are dressed more formally than usual. None wear gloves, since there is no cutting in the cadavers today; indeed students are not even permitted to touch the exhibits. It is also the first cool day this fall (it's raining steadily), so shorts are uncommon. Possibly some have used dressing and grooming rituals as a source of confidence; there's more make-up among the women, and long hair, usually covered or put up for anatomy lab, is down. As Lisa told me, pulling on her long, taffy-colored hair, "You can put it up and get it out of the way all right, but the stupid fumes still get in it. I always go home and wash my hair, right after lab." Even the informal Jonathan has complained, "You always feel dirty after lab."

The promised "tour guide" is Dr. English himself, meeting each group at the appointed elevator. He gives instructions and gets in at least one joke: "Do not write on the exam, even if you feel compelled to write 'Great Question!" he exhorts. He leads the students to the twenty-five stations (twenty-two tagged cadavers, two X rays, and a thoracic vertebra on a tray) as well as "rest stations"—three or four extra yellow chairs (depending on the number of students per group). English gets everyone positioned and yells, "Okay, start!" One of the lab coordinators runs a timer that gives electronic tones every seventy-five seconds, when the students must move to the next station, carrying their answer sheets in hand. Each station contains the exhibit in the cadaver (a tagged nerve, muscle, blood vessel, or bone), the typed-out question with five choices, a pencil, and a copy of the entire exam, so that the student can look back to check anything; all these rest on a book rack. A lab instructor stands in the hall, available to help a student.

"Help!" one calls out, and the white-coated instructor runs up the hall, aware that the student has only so many seconds for that answer. I peek into the room—it's the Outpost—and see a single vertebra on a white tray. Apparently the last student through picked up the bone—despite the prohibition against touching—and put it down the wrong way, hiding the tag. The instructor turns the bone over. I keep an eye on the room and learn that about half the students pick it up.

I watch the students move from station to station. Most mark their answers quickly, since the problem is clear, the five choices contain the right answer, and, evidently, the students are well prepared. In the big rooms, at least, they are careful not to touch anything: they lean over exhibits and bend to the side in exaggerated postures of attention. Many hold their hands with the answer sheet behind them, looking vaguely like white chickens. Here and there are the students I recognize from Room 1, now resolutely working their way through this obstacle course.

One of the women bends over the cadaver, peering intently; her beautiful long brown hair falls forward around her cheeks. With one hand she gathers her locks and holds them at her throat. Her gaze focuses on whatever structure is labeled below. She's Miss Y, whose good looks are well known among the M-1 men, at least the ones I have heard gossiping about their female classmates. My guess is that the guys would envy the cadaver inches below her face. The contrast is remarkable: a vital young woman in the flush of health versus a corpse with its chest and abdomen cut open. Perhaps her beauty is especially compelling if we see the corpse as a *memento mori*; someday—far in the future, I hope—her body will be equally dead.

In forty minutes the group is done and charging down the other set of stairs, as the next group gathers. After the last group has finished the exam, I take a quick tour through the stations, finding everything neatly tagged and the lamps set so that each exhibit is brightly lit. The circumstances for the "gaze" have a clear focus here; either you know the answer or you don't. At the same time, I can see how students would want to pick up that vertebra; so much of their learning has been tactile, it must be hard to shift to looking only.

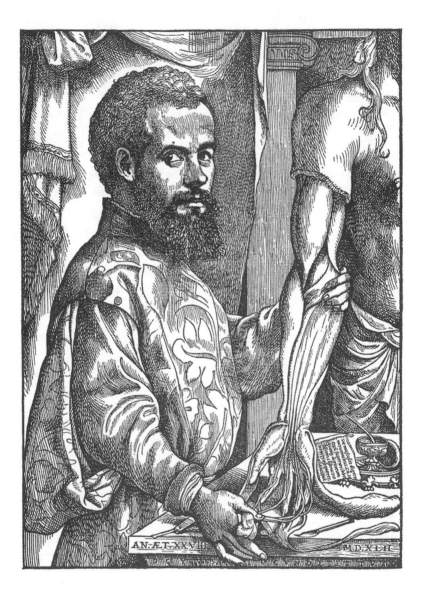

REPORTS I'VE READ consider this formal portrait of Vesalius to be fairly accurate, even including a birthmark or wart above his right eyebrow. Here, he poses in his finest clothes, as if at work, showing how tendons insert into fingers and cause them to grasp. A scalpel lies on the table and, behind it, an ink pot and some writing, which starts *"de musculis digitorum . . ."* ("concerning the muscles of the fingers . . ."). Like most anatomists until about ten years ago, he does not use gloves.

On the table's edge we read that Vesalius was twenty-eight, and that the portrait was done in 1442. Below this, letters obscurely appear: *"ocyus, iuncunde et tuto,"* or, according to Saunders and O'Malley, " 'swiftly, pleasantly, and safely' —a motto apparently derived from an aphorism of the ancient physician Asclepiades," referring to how a physician should heal a patient (page 41).

This woodcut affords a rare view of a cadaver partially dissected so that we can see, on the upper arm, the layer of fat just under the skin. The cadaver's loins are modestly draped. How it is supported is not clear.

CUTTING WITH VESALIUS

· · ·

(FIRST ESSAY)

I N ANATOMICAL LANGUAGE, "reflection" is the physical turning back of
large structures, such as skin flaps or muscles, so that the underlying parts
can be seen. Over the last few weeks the students have so often asked me
whether I'd take their laboratory exam that I began to feel the need for some
kind of reflective examination, even in the monastic isolation of my library
study. I think a self-directed exercise will help me step back from the lectures, texts, and dissections of the course to consider underlying patterns
and meanings. Not a necessity but a heuristic, my game is in some ways parallel to the students' lab exam—an obstacle course that both tests and creates knowledge.

A book lover by habit, by calling, I start my inquiry by turning to a book,
the sixteenth-century anatomy by Vesalius introduced earlier in the course,
De humani corporis fabrica (On the Fabric of the Human Body). To see an original copy of this treasure, I must take the elevator to the top floor of Emory
University's Robert W. Woodruff Library for Advanced Studies, which
houses the Special Collections Department. The librarian asks me to fill out
forms and to "show a picture ID." Care must be taken with a book worth upward of $20,000.

The book comes from the stacks in a large, protective cardboard box. The volume was rebound in 1949 in a neutral but handsome leather binding. I am required to leave all pens behind; only pencils are allowed in the reading room. The librarian doesn't hand the work directly to me but sets up large wedges of gray sponge rubber ("book supports") on the table, making a stand. This arrangement protects the binding and puts the book in a convenient slant, reminiscent of medieval desks. The book is physically imposing, about sixteen inches high, eight inches wide, three inches thick. The librarian opens the book to the middle and says, "Here you are."

Published in 1543, *De fabrica* is exactly 400 years older than I am. I turn the big pages with reverence; the paper is high quality, solid-feeling, but pliable. The printing is crisp. It has been said that Gutenberg not only invented printing (in the West), but that he perfected it, because his model was fine calligraphy. Printed in Basel about 100 years after Gutenberg's Bibles, Vesalius's revolutionary work came at a strategic time for wide distribution: it was one of the early books spread by the new mass medium of printing.

In the thirty-two-page index, I find over 200 references to Galen, the great classical authority (and physician to the ailing, stoic Marcus Aurelius). I look up some of these references and find deferential but corrective language, as best as my Latin can make out. (I read elsewhere that Vesalius's Latin was "extremely corrupt" and difficult to translate; apparently no one has rendered this huge book into English.) Vesalius pays homage to Galen, calling him "easily the chief of the professors of dissection," but also points out "that he himself never dissected the body of a man who had recently died." Vesalius became the founder of modern anatomy. Previous cutters avoided human bodies (sometimes by religious decree), relied on animals for dissection, and/or assumed that Galen was always correct. Vesalius rejected animals, used human cadavers, and did not hesitate to correct Galen when his observations differed.

I look at the portrait of Vesalius and see, near him, his scalpel looking much the same as those the students use, although a single piece of metal, not with a detachable blade. I think of all the cutting this man must have done to gain the knowledge shown here, the observation, the reconciliation of variations in human beings, and the work with the artist(s) who put his knowledge into wonderful clarity through another kind of cutting, incising wood for woodcuts. I turn every one of the 750 pages of the book, out of reverence for the writer and engravers who created this masterpiece. It is divided into seven books, on bones, muscles, blood vessels, nerves, the abdominal viscera, the thoracic viscera, and—although not well understood in Renaissance times—the brain. The paragraphs pile up, the woodcuts—scores of them—lead the eye on.

Suddenly Vesalius becomes for me the presiding genius of the anatomy lab a few buildings away. Since modern methods often follow his methods, his woodcuts show very well what the med students are doing in their lab this semester. As they cut there, they take up a 400-year-old tradition and make it more and more their own. The anatomy lab, at first a forbidding and remote place, increasing becomes familiar to them, a precursor to many rooms they will pursue their life's work in: clinics, emergency rooms, operating rooms, hospital rooms. Eventually they will be able to read bodies as easily as they read books, as I turn the pages of this one.

The students have been cutting and looking for four weeks now, gaining the knowledge that allows them to answer exam questions, while the cadavers become more ragged, with various parts now in plastic bags. I have been musing over the strange relationship of cutting in order to construct knowledge, of destroying in order to build an understanding of the body. Part of my self-exam, then, should focus on this concept of cutting. To "cut" is the essence of anatomical activity. The students say, "Are you cutting this afternoon?" Their instrument cases are full of tools that slice, scissor, puncture, poke, or tear. They learn to use the handles for "blunt" dissection, and even their own fingers to divide tissues. One way or another, one living body cuts into a dead body. The very word *anatomy* comes from the Greek (*ana,* "up"; *tomy,* from *temnein,* "to cut"). An "appendectomy" means the cutting (out) of the appendix. (Even a "tome," or book, was originally a "cut," as from a roll of papyrus.) In the parallel ancient language, Latin, *secare* means "to cut," the root for several medical words and phrases: *dissection,* bowel *resection,* cesarean *section.* Cutting separates either one organ from another or parts of one organ (the heart, say) from itself. The job of anatomical cutting is to clarify the structure and function of these tissues.

Cutting, in its wider, metaphoric sense, is remarkably Western, an ancient philosophical and scientific concept. Democritus wanted to find atoms (*a,* "not"; *tom,* "cuttable"), the absolute, tiny building blocks for the cuttable universe. Aristotle was a "splitter" who cut categories apart, each with their own set of causes. Texts called anatomies appeared for bodies and soon, metaphorically, for many other subjects. Burton's *Anatomy of Melancholy,* for example, is a massive, four-volume discussion of one of the notorious illnesses of the seventeenth century. Near the same time, Descartes joined (and intensified) this tradition with his divisions of subject and object, as well as mind and matter. The rise of modern science, the industrial revolution, computers, and the cyberworld owe much to these separations and divisions; to "anatomize" something has come to mean, intellectually, to divide and conquer. Northrop Frye's modern book of literary theory, *Anatomy of Criticism,* shrewdly (and elliptically) carries no article: neither "an" anatomy (one way of doing it) nor "the" anatomy (a peremptory claim), but perhaps an action or activity, suggesting the ongoing process of dividing and ordering. Norman Cousins called the account of his illness and recovery *Anatomy of an Illness,* even though one of his themes is the need for synthesis in health matters, not endless anatomizing.

Indeed, one of the debates in contemporary Western medicine concerns the challenge to see the human body as an integration of materials, ideas, emotions, and spirit, all within social relationships (the so-called biopsychosocial model). Much criticism of modern Western medicine sees it as too technical, too limited, too reductive of what a human being actually is. In the anatomy lab students are seeing more and more of each cadaver unwrapped, inviting them to think more and more about them as remains of human beings, not just lab exhibits. While the dissections still emphasize particular areas of the body and salient structures, the students are increasingly interested in the past life of their cadavers and how the whole thing "goes together."

To cut is also to make space, to separate matter so that light can enter, eyes may see. In anatomy, "potential space" is a phrase that refers, for example, to the two pleural linings around the lungs. Ordinarily they stick together, so that when the chest rises it pulls the lungs upward and outward, creating the partial vacuum that causes air to enter the lungs. If a stab wound introduces air into the chest, however, these layers may separate, making an actual space so that the lung won't rise. This is a condition known as pneumothorax; if there is blood filling the space, it is hemothorax (what Ronald Reagan suffered when he was shot). Another example of potential space is the vagina, ordinarily closed in folds, appearing on cross-section as the letter H, or so I have read. For intercourse or birth, this potential space becomes actual. In the discipline of anatomy, however, any body part, whether an organ, a muscle, or even a bone, can be seen as potential space, since cutting is the actualizer, making space for the gaze: to see, to learn, to name. Any potential space might be seen symbolically like the vagina, a birth canal for the emergence of knowledge. For the ancient Greeks, maieutics was the art of aiding in childbirth. The anatomy lab, we might say, is a maieutic place, a womb where knowledge is birthed, and the students, with scalpels or probes in hand, are midwives of a sort to their own learning.

The living human body has weight, volume, multidimensionality. The only ways into its spaces are through ordinary orifices relating to air, food, and sex, or through harmful cuts: wounds. For cadavers, by contrast, cuts are not wounds, but inquisitive gestures, pointed questions (so to speak), or even compliments. There are shy cuts and bold cuts, brief cuts and extended cuts, cuts light as a caress or decisive as a duelist's. Despite these differences, they are all epistemological, all seeking knowledge within the natural order of bodies. This nature, or *phusis* in the Greek term, becomes the business of the *physician:* to know the body's parts, their functions, their relations in sickness and in health.

But while we may speak of the anatomy of a flower, a movie actress, or a fetal pig, the true anatomy is not the structure of those actual objects, that material per se, but the *discipline,* the activity, the intellectual approach that leads to a comprehensive and synthetic wisdom. And much of this emerges from (or at least starts with) the *-tomy,* the cutting. This cutting shows (and, in a sense, *creates,* by providing consciousness and words) the physical structures. We are not talking about random cutting, or the anatomy course would be over in a few hours of slashing. Nor is it mutilation, through which the symbolic worth of the body is lost; the discipline of anatomy, rightly pursued, provides order, validation, and affirmation, even as the bodies slowly come apart, disintegrating toward chaos. The students I watch seem profoundly touched by the intricacy and majesty of the human body as they painstakingly work their way through it.

The students cut because they must, but also because they have chosen this training. So far, in this first third of the course, I have seen among the students three general responses to the cadaver. Initially, for many there is disgust and aversion. Typically (but not always) these responses soon fade away, as they did for Jonathan and Steve. Next is the reduction of the cadaver to a biological exhibit through draping, through a tight physical focus (one area of the back, say), and through an understanding of cutting (or the discipline of anatomy) as the main mode of perception and interpretation. Finally, as the course goes on, the cadaver itself seems to break through these attempts at reduction to reassert its own humanity, by presenting oddities, intricacies, and variations; so far Nero is the best example of this "rehumanization," because his torso is distinctly different from the others in its bulk. Although the hair is clipped to make the cadavers "generic," the irrepressible individuality of each body becomes clear anyway, as a particular body of a particular sex that belonged to an actual person with a human history. When students begin to roam from table to table and from room to room, they gain a wider sense of bodies in general, varieties of bodies, and *the human body* that is the basic home for all human life.

As the students make their way through much demanding handiwork, their confidence grows. They find—despite their fears—the structures required for identification by the syllabus. They do "clean dissections," which earn them good grades. They are not punished by Nemesis for removing the heart from a body. Cutting slowly becomes less an alien activity and more just one of the jobs for the week, however exacting and tedious. And as the cutting becomes much easier technically, they can better enjoy (even *appreciate*) the complexity and variety of the human bodies before them. As the students visit among tables to compare and to learn, the cutting becomes more social, less an individual and lonely activity; they meet more bodies, both alive and dead.

What are the purposes and models for cutting? At base, there is a common purpose: to learn about the body, its parts, their names, and their relations. For the practice of medicine—at least in the Western tradition—knowing the parts and their relations is a *sine qua non,* the foundation for everything else that follows. To know basic human anatomy is to have the blueprint, the map, the globe: an in-depth familiarity with the very habitus of health or the lack of health. While physicians have various offices and hospitals to practice in, their constant workbench is this human body.

Further, there is the reliance on the authority of the various models that serve as guides, most prominently words and drawings. The drawings are of many kinds: engravings, schematic drawings, color prints, slides, even paper models (see Figure 14 below), but also X rays, CT scans, and sonograms; in each case the illustrator (or technician) seeks to use line, tone, and/or color to give an accurate rendition of the structures of the body. Such models, while clarifying in some sense, always distort in others: three dimensions become two; colors become shades of gray. In the late 1970s a facsimile 1901 edition of *Gray's Anatomy* suddenly and unexpectedly became a bestseller, even though its Victorian prose, packed with scientific words, is difficult to read. It was popular not because of the text but because, I think, the book was a symbol of understanding and control of the body, particularly through the elegant (but inevitably simplifying) engravings. At some level, we yearn to understand, to know in depth, to control these bodies we live in. Part of the attraction of the anatomy lab for me is to see the complex and interweaving structures of the body clarified by pictures and language.

There are thousands of specialized anatomical terms that have been subjects of international debate. Greek, Roman, and Arab scientists (and still others) advanced name upon name, until there were some 50,000, many overlapping, according to a congress of anatomists in 1895. After deliberation, modern anatomists chose mostly Latin terms and reduced the number to about 5,000, which are the basis for today's vocabulary (now expanded to about 6,500, according to the *Nomina anatomica* revised in Mexico City in 1980). Medical students must learn a portion of this nomenclature, its pronunciations, and pervasive roots (like *-tomy*) that are universal among scientists. Outsiders have parodied this jargon; one example is the supposed gynecologist's greeting: "At your cervix, madam; dilated to meet you." The students have their own slang ("a real bitch," "cadaver juice") even as they learn to say "obturator," "splanchnic," and "postganglionic."

The students are also building a method, an understanding of some of the basic ways the body works. Given a muscle, for example, the students can study its attachments and frame a reasonable idea about the movement caused by its contracture. The instructors for this course emphasize problem solving, even in the frame for the ten-minute presentations. Anatomy, as a discipline of thought, slowly assembles in the students' minds as a resource—an armature—for much of their future training.

There is a final concept, briefly introduced the first day but reinforced by every visit of the chaplain: that the anatomical work proceeds within some "larger dimensions." The tight focus of anatomical dissection might become an excuse to avoid such awareness, but the claim, from the beginning, that there are values beyond just finding and naming stays as a counterpoint to the formal course. The students know that the Service of Reflection and Gratitude will close the semester, and this goal helps them keep wider notions in mind.

If such are the purposes and methods for cutting by anatomy students, what are mine? How does a humanist cut? As a student, I used to buy cheap French editions that were sold "uncut"; these books were bound so that the edges and the top of the pages folded over to other pages: you could not read the book without first cutting through these folds. (A true gentleman would send such books to his printer, for trimming and binding in full morocco—or whatever.) For us lesser folks it became part of the tactile ritual of reading to slice open the pages in their repeating patterns, storing the knife in the book as a bookmark. Perhaps any book is a "potential space" for the activity of our minds, something like a playground or a dance floor. Or is it the other way around, that our minds are the potential space for the book to jump and dance? Either way—or both—the act of cutting emphasized the active role of the reader in the opening up of a book's meanings. This particular delight has disappeared from my life (does anyone still do this? I wonder), but it serves as a metaphor for the opening of all books, including Vesalius's magnum opus, and even embalmed bodies. The anatomy course teaches reading of the texts of dead bodies; whether encountering a book of poems or a human heart, the reader's hand and eye provide information to our interpreting brains.

My perceptions of the "book of the lab" are largely guided by the students, as I look over their shoulders and listen to what they say. Our points of view are starting to diverge, however, since they are rapidly outstripping me in knowledge of anatomy, and I know now that I will never become a physician. I'm discovering that I'd rather write about health and medicine than follow these studies or attempt to do clinical work. I'd prefer to arrange words, images, and stories that describe and interpret. Students and I both ruminate upon the vivid stimuli of the lab and our responses, making inquiry and moving toward analysis and interpretation. The students' focus, of course, is the memorization and analysis that will serve them on their exams; my interpretations are in a different direction and are just becoming clear to me. Finally, we each make our own synthesis, whether a ten-minute presentation or a manuscript of scores of pages.

A cantaloupe vine—like the students, the cadavers, and the lab instructors—has also been my teacher through these weeks of late summer. When my wife and I were moving into our apartment for the year, we parked the rented truck as close as possible to our building but still had to walk around (or through—depending on our patience) a large bed of marigolds. In the midst of these, there was a weedy vine. By what accident had a seed taken root here? A passing bird? The next day, I looked at it more closely and found three cantaloupes attached, two fist-sized, one grocery store–sized. Over the next two weeks, I kept an eye on this volunteer vine and its produce, figuring someone would pick the melon and take it inside, but no one did. One day, I found the melon detached, and an insect inspecting the place where the vine previously attached, presumably the best point of entry. The insect sought to be, in its own fashion, a cutter. With the insect's help, the sun, and various bacteria, the melon would rot, providing nourishment for its many seeds, some of which might bear fruit in their own season.

Neither the insect nor the sun would have this fruit, however; I brushed the insect away and took the melon inside to chill in the refrigerator. My wife and I ate it for breakfast; it tasted good. How did the fruit know when to fall off the vine? How did it "cut" itself loose? What complex timings are there for any departures from life? For the turn of the seasons? To what purpose? These are, of course, ancient questions. John quotes Jesus saying, "Truly, truly, I say to you, unless a grain of wheat falls to the earth and dies, it remains alone; but if it dies, it bears much fruit" (John 12: 24, R.S.V.). André Gide was captivated by this paradox and entitled his autobiographical memoir after it, *Se le grain ne meurt,* usually translated *If It Die.* From death comes new life.

I begin to think of the cadavers in the anatomy lab as fruits that separated from life, in their own season, each by their own internal necessity. I think of the dead in my family, especially those who died young, including my father. I hope their time was, somehow, right. The med students benefit from the maturity of the cadavers, their ripeness. For everything there is a season, we read in Ecclesiastes, a time to be born, and a time to die. Somehow a cantaloupe seed took root among the marigolds. Somehow each of us appears on earth, children of our parents' egg and seed. And all that is planted eventually dies. Somehow nineteen cadavers, ripe and harvested fruit, are now in this anatomy lab. They are here as fabulous texts, whole libraries of wisdom, ready for the inspection of 113 students, whose cuts are the plowings and plantings that create new knowledge.

．　．　．

It is early autumn now in Georgia, the time for fruits to ripen and, soon, leaves to fall. Somehow I am lucky enough to be here, to look, to witness. The students cut in the tradition of Vesalius, and I look over their shoulders. We each cut in different ways, and all of us are increasingly able to see more within these bodies and within ourselves, deepening our own humanity while studying the unusual humanity of the dead.

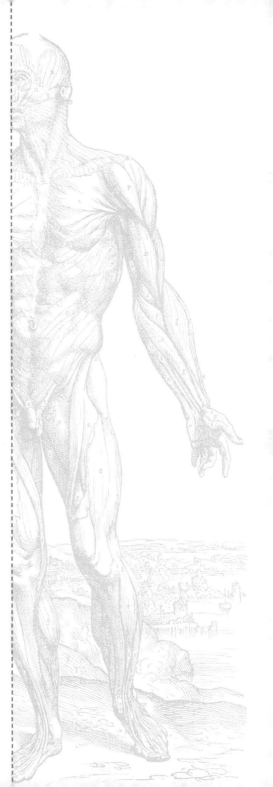

PART II

INTO INTIMACIES

Muscles of the Pelvic Cavity

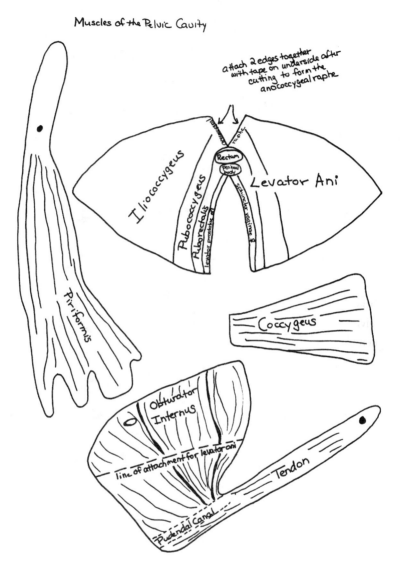

THE MUSCLES OF THE PELVIC CAVITY

(Figure 14)

THESE FOUR SHAPES represent, in paper-doll fashion, various muscles of the pelvic floor. Students are encouraged to cut these from the syllabus and fit them into the bones of the articulated skeleton.

(Design by Barbara Brown, Ph.D.; from *Human Anatomy Course Syllabus,* 1989, Emory University, following page 92. Used by permission).

WE GOT A LADY, REMEMBER?

• • •

H EY, HOWARD, YOU want to hear our presentation?" I'm hearing this routinely now, as students recite to me, to each other, to the smelly air of the lab if no one will listen. They show the bony landmarks on the skeleton, trace the muscles covering the abdomen, show the nerves, pull back the flaps, and display the abdominal contents, still more or less in place. Through the students, flesh is made word.

David and Cliff are sure they'll be next to last to present and don't even uncover the cadaver. Besides, there's much discussion of the laboratory exam, particularly the key posted in the hall, which verifies which guesses turned out felicitously. Complains one student: "Damn, you don't get any credit for knowing enough to throw out three choices if you guess wrong between the remaining two!" Another student worries that she gave her group wrong information from her dissection: "Did I lead us all astray on that question? I checked it with the lab instructor, even." I learn that no one failed either part of the exam, although several wish they had done better. "I guess I'll have to study a bit harder," I hear a few saying. One man says, "It really wasn't that hard if you had studied enough—which I think I'll try next time."

Despite the varying levels of success, all students are relieved to have the exam over. They carry more stuff—books, backpacks, jackets—into the lab: they are moving in. HAPPY BIRTHDAY KAREN is written on the blackboard.

As we start the middle third of the course, the anatomy lab is less an alien place, and something more like home.

The lab instructor finally comes to Table 3, and Cliff and David go into their spiels. This is their third time around, and they seem quite comfortable. I have asked them for permission to listen, so I stand closer than usual. They do fine, running through the structures, relations, and terminology. At one point Cliff pulls up David's shirt to show where organs are beneath the external landmarks. There's considerable joking and laughter among the people watching at this sudden unveiling of David's pale abdomen, even to the point that Cliff slows down and falters. David's poker face is solemn and studious while Cliff probes his stomach, but the hilarity in the room crescendos until the methodical Cliff cracks up with laughter. He stops a moment and adjusts his glasses. The instructor acknowledges this delay by giving extra time when her timer goes off at ten minutes. She likes the presentation, though, and awards them a good grade; they leave with smiles on their faces.

What kind of doctors will David and Cliff be? One of the qualities I see in David is calmness, a still center that would be comforting to me as a distraught patient. Certainly this quality would be welcome in many fields, but I think particularly of psychiatry and any field with chronic illness—for which patients and families need continuous support. And Cliff? His passion seems acutely intellectual, as he compares models and exhibits, books and bodies, ideas and actualities. As long as guessing is free, I'll imagine him solving problems in internal medicine or medical research. Maybe he could figure out the cancer that killed my father.

"And here we go again, as clueless as before!" I hear behind me. It's Steve and, shortly, Jonathan. They complain about being tired and unprepared, but as they begin cutting, they snap their scalpel blades on smoothly and dig right in.

"I'll read, you cut," declares Jonathan, but shortly they are both deep into the abdomen, cutting, dividing, tracing. Jonathan uses his gloved hands to separate the gallbladder from the surrounding tissues. "Hey, this thing's full of gravel!" he calls out. At Jonathan's invitation I feel the green sac and the little stones rolling around inside like buckshot: it is packed with gallstones. "Did this give her pain, you think?" they ask the lab instructor when he passes by. "Very possibly not," he replied. "Lots of people carry gallstones asymptomatically."

Jonathan uses his fingers to separate this green bladder from the liver. "Nice going," says Steve. Steve dissects blood vessels free at the top of the abdomen. Jonathan is separating bowels lower down.

"I am thoroughly enjoying this now, Steven," he chuckles.

Around the room, the talk is direct.

"Hey, can we see your colon?"

"This stomach is just like a wine sack."

"Where does the celiac artery go?"

"I kind of like to play with guts. Look how they settle back into place all by themselves."

There is also a kind of group conversation around the room unknown in previous weeks. The hushed atmosphere is gone; students call and visit from table to table, sticking their heads close to the opened abdomens to compare, to make sure they're on the right track.

One woman calls out, "Did you hear what happened to Lex?"

"What happened?"

"Well, he was trimming out some fat with his head down close, you know, and a bit flipped out and went right into his mouth."

"No!"

"Really! And he ran to the sink to spit it out and to wash his mouth out."

"Oooooo!"

"We asked him what it tasted like, and he said he tried not to taste it."

Another topic is the departure of one of their fellow first-year medical students. "So we're a hundred and twelve strong, now," is one formulation. The students I hear are supportive of his decision, understanding it as a reasonable choice. I ask them how they feel about their chances of making it through. "Well, we should be all set. *Pre*-med's really the worst," Larry at Table 1 explains. "The dean here told us when we got here that ninety-eight percent will graduate. And the other two percent usually make the choice to leave the program." Others nod in assent, and I realize that they view themselves as "having made it" in a sense: if they do the work, they'll be doctors.

This attitude contrasts with the traditional tales of med school. The grayhaired dean would welcome the first-years with, "Look on your left . . . and on your right. One of these persons will not graduate, since our completion rate is fifty percent." Those days are gone. Now, if you're *on the track,* you'll make it. Why? There are several reasons: a higher number of applications (8,000 applications yielding 800 interviews for 100 spots at some schools) ensures a higher quality of student; learning models have changed from Darwinian competition to cooperative learning, and, of course, the commonsensical notion that med schools invest a lot of money in each graduate and feel, therefore, a greater responsibility to get an entire class through their studies to the M.D. degree.

Two countermotifs enrich the afternoon. The first is satiric, a listing of "rules" on the blackboard. These make up an ironic commentary much in the tradition of *The House of God,* a sarcastic novel that has been a favorite of medical students since it came out in 1978. Steve scrawls the first rule, chalk splintering and flying with his energy:

RULE #1 IF IT BREAKS IT WASN'T IMPORTANT

Immediately another student races up to the board to make his contribution:

RULE #2 WING IT

Another hand adds:

RULE #3 IT CAN'T LOOK LIKE THE PICTURE

Immediate laughter validates these insights, both as satiric vengeance and as a kind of community building. The rules are practical, as well. The students have learned that the cadavers rarely look exactly like the picture; they are now careful to look at several cadavers to create their own sense of norms and variations.

The second countermotif involves a discovery in the next room, reputed to be a steel tank full of heads. Saeed, from Table 2, leads little tours, declaring that sight to be "weird." I take my turn, following him over for a look, and we stop by an enclosed tank. He assures me again that it is weird but makes no effort to lift the lid. I open the lid and see immediately a floating head with orange eyes wide open; they appear to be staring directly at me. This vision is so arresting that I can't really "see" anything else in the box, although I'm aware that other things are bobbing in the clear liquid. I lower the lid.

"Yes, certainly weird," I manage.

Just about everyone in the first room makes the trip. By contrast, our cadavers seem like old friends. But the urge to see something *beyond,* no matter how strange, seems to be an important motivator in this anatomical work.

Steve and Jonathan have settled into a natural division of labor. Steve is working the descending blood vessels free as they pass through the diaphragm. He first dissects from above, then from below. Suddenly his fingers have penetrated this large domed muscle that separates the chest cavity from the abdomen.

"Whoopee," he calls out. "Look at my fingers!" We admire his gloved fingers wiggling in the space where the heart used to be. The diaphragm, crucial to breathing, was thought by the ancient Greeks to be the seat of the soul and, later, the soul itself.

Jonathan cuts on the lower end, following the descending colon down over the bony rim that defines the beginning of the pelvic cavity. "I'm really getting down to the *root* of things," he announces. As he pushes intestines up to get them out of his way, they push the omentum—a fatty apron covering the bowels—up into Steve's area.

"Hey, get this omentum outta my face!" he protests.

"Ooops, sorry."

I look out the window and muse about Steve and Jonathan as physicians. I can see Jonathan possibly as a sports physician, backslapping and joking with bruising (and bruised) behemoths, while Steve, ever alert and expressive, might he become a doctor for children? Surely my speculations are facile, and while such roles are certainly plausible, dozens of others are equally likely, and the good humor and affability of both men will be strong resources in whatever specialty they practice.

"Holy moly," Jonathan says, "what is this stuff?" The men look into the pelvic cavity to see a smooth knob between two bands of connective tissue.

"Hey, it's the uterus! We got a lady, remember?"

"Right, and here's an ovary," a bean-shaped structure projecting into the cavity from the side, like a little ear.

"With the uterine tube leading down."

They look and are silent for a moment. It's a moment of reverence: the cadaver becomes deeper, fuller to them. Did this woman have children? What is it like to carry a child? Did she enjoy sex? Can this little, pink knob really create babies? Was that truly the first home for every one of us?

In a moment they resume work, but show their discoveries to anyone passing by.

"Hey, Mark, did you find your ovaries? Look in here!"

Mark peers in. "That's the genuine article, I'd say. Of course, if we find them, we'll be in big trouble."

"Why's that?"

"Our cadaver is a male."

EASIER TO FIND
THAN TO NAME
· · ·

HOW'S IT GOING, Steve?" He is seated on a stool over at the counter area, picking fat from a mound of guts in front of him. He and Jonathan were in last night to remove the entire abdominal *en bloc,* as anatomists like to say, although there is assuredly not a hard right angle anywhere in this mess. Steve pokes at the heap of guts, stomach, liver, and pancreas that sprawls before him on a white enamel tray.

"Oh, I'm finding all sorts of stuff, nerves, veins, arteries," he says. "But which ones are they? It's easier to find than to name these things."

It's a complex dissection, especially with the viscera away from their bony landmarks, sprawling and slithering according to gravity. But it's also complicated for the other students working on the remaining wreck of the torso. With lungs and heart gone from the chest and the abdominal contents removed, the diaphragm hangs like a rag in the large space. The jagged ribs stick up at the sides, appearing something like a shipwreck.

Jonathan peers in. "What are you?" he bellows into the cavity. "Speak up!"

The students now recognize structures as veins, arteries, nerves, ligaments, but they are further required to know them in order and by name. Scott vows to create a plastic cadaver with every part labeled. "It'll cost forty thousand dollars, but it'll be worth it." He and his partner have started their own model, in chalk on the blackboard above the cadaver, a schematic listing of blood vessels. "Yep, we've found all of those," he tells me.

Back in the first room, the labeling question becomes a topic for group conversation.

"Maybe if there were buttons in the cadaver. You push the button on the structure and get the name."

"Yeah, like in a museum."

"Or a national park."

"I'd settle for a computer, right here at the side." The conversation continues, revealing a hunger for names, order, connections of theory and concrete body parts. The underlying and eventual solution, of course, is in the mind of each student, where the computer, the buttons, the model is slowly being assembled.

"Look at this beautiful pancreatic duct," Steve calls out. The pancreas, a floppy, conical finger, is not intrinsically one of the more beautiful organs. Its name means "all flesh," and it looks like something to be thrown out. It is the offending organ in an early chapter of Sinclair Lewis's *Arrowsmith,* when high-spirited medical students place a pancreas into the hat of the trustee, as he strolls around the lab, holding his hat behind him. Nonetheless, the organ is important biologically, providing insulin and glucagon for the body; when it fails, diabetes mellitus is one of the diseases that can result.

Shortly Steve says, "I'm going to close this puppy up and go read a while. I need some more terms." He takes his anatomy books down to a room full of plastic models and sits at a desk, poring over pictures and text. Back in the lab, Cliff drops by to watch Jonathan cut and to look at the anatomy text on the book rack. It's a colored atlas, the sort initially scorned by Jonathan and Steve. One photograph of abdominal organs is wonderfully clear, with photos of arteries and veins injected with colored latex. The terms are printed to the side, linked to the structures with straight lines. Cliff is excited at this view, and guesses, usually accurately, what the structures are before looking at the identifications.

Today, the most dramatic series of events is at Nero's table. Nero, immense as ever, lies under his white coverings. Kathy is alone today, since her partner is at an unavoidable meeting. She unwraps the hulk. Most of the other tables are ahead of her, many with the viscera already out. "Well, you'll have more space than the rest of us, once you get that Gargantua disemboweled," one student calls from across the room. "Thanks a lot," she replies, pondering the mountain in front of her.

As students lift the contents out of the Fatless Man, Kathy says, "Is that *all* you have from him?" "That's it; neat, huh?" they reply. Their load, remarkably clean of fat, is probably only one-third of what she will excavate from Nero. Fat is a big topic today, since it is a prime obstacle to the dissection. At Table 5, the conversation turns to buffalo kidney fat, reputed to be a prime cookstuff for certain American Indians.

Fortunately, Mike (Team A) comes in to give Kathy a hand, and one of the lab instructors helps make some cuts and plan some strategy. It takes all three of them to handle Nero's guts. As the organs become more disconnected from the cavity, Mike, fearful that they will cascade onto him at his side of the table, cries out, "Hey, don't avalanche me!"

Soon Kathy announces: "The bowel from hell is about to come out." Mike calls for music. They heave and pull the stuff onto a tray laid across Nero's groin.

"Damn, one tray isn't going to be enough!" one says.

Back at Table 3, Jonathan is working hesitantly at the psoas muscle deep in the pelvis. Visiting from the next room, Mark says, "You gotta get that out of there to find the nerves," but Jonathan worries about cutting important structures below. Then Dr. Richard Margeson (a local surgeon who donates time to the training of young physicians) looks in.

"What do we have here?" he asks, automatically adjusting the light for the best illumination; some students still don't even turn theirs on.

"I guess I need to get through this psoas muscle," Jonathan says.

"Yes, well let's see here. . . ." The silver-haired Dr. Margeson pulls from his lab-coat pocket two instruments. One is a forceps (long tongs) and the other a pair of surgical scissors with short blades but very long handles. Since these instruments are about twelve inches long, Dr. Margeson appears to be working by remote control, his gloveless hands well above the cadaver.

Below, the stainless steel flashes in the light. The instruments work together smoothly, as if they were a pair of metallic ballet dancers. He separates with the forceps and cuts with the scissors. Sometimes he cuts with the scissors as anyone might, but now and then he inserts them with the blades closed, then opens them to spread tissues. Several of us watch spellbound. The psoas muscle neatly, relentlessly—but somehow deliberately—comes apart, and important structures are separated out, undamaged. Evidently, these are the moves of a master surgeon.

"Wow, those scissors are great!" someone says.

"That's like saying McEnroe's racket is great," Margeson quips; the students chuckle. The man who praised the scissors shuffles his feet. Dr. Margeson slides the instruments into his pocket and goes to wash his hands.

"Do you *know* what just happened here?" Jonathan says with wonder.

"Tell me."

"That man saved me over an hour! What an animal. . . . I was too timid. What an animal!"

Besides his size, the other unmistakable quality about Nero is that he smells. All the cadavers smell, of course, but mostly of formaldehyde. Nero smells like, well, rotting meat. Various cutters have commented on this since just after Labor Day, five weeks ago. During this time, his odor has gotten worse. On the advice of a lab instructor, Mike and Kathy decide to wash out his abdominal cavity with liquid soap. They pull the rubber hose over from the sinks and view the cavern below.

"We gotta fill up this birdbath," Mike mutters and orders me to stand on the pedals that run both the hot and cold water. Mike extends the green hose and aims the stream of water into the cavity, as if watering a strange flower box. I imagine meaty flowers growing up (indeed, the word *carnation* implies meat), anatomical bouquets for the students to sniff and admire—and explain.

NOT MUCH ROOM IN THERE

· · ·

ATELY I'VE BEEN hearing some trepidation about the upcoming dissection of the pelvis and its contents. The usual formulation is something like, "There's not much room in there; I don't see how two of us are going to work." While it is a small volume of space to work in—as opposed to the chest and the abdomen—there are more than just mechanical concerns: the genitals have at least as much symbolic power as the heart, which provoked much anxiety a few weeks back.

Students can talk pretty openly about the face and the hands, now that they're more comfortable with these parts. "I've got a friend at another med school," one tells me. "They start with the face, shred that up, and then treat the rest of the cadaver as a sheep or dog or something. They even cut the whole thing in half!" But the genitals have not been much discussed—except for a few joking references—and they have been kept covered. This relatively small area is saturated not only with nerves and blood vessels, but, of course, with value-laden meanings and emotions.

The lectures on the pelvic region seem to have a certain fascination. Dr. English has a nice joke in one of the slides that shows the trip a sperm takes from the testes, through the body, out the penile urethra to the "outside (or inside) world." The students all laugh. English explains that he can't take credit, since his wife prepared the slide. Further appreciative laughter. The dice for this dissection are clearly loaded, and these young women and men are as full of vital juices as anyone.

There is more anxious talk as we head upstairs. One students says, "Well, I gotta go put on the greasy shirt." Others are quoting to each other from the syllabus: " 'Force the feet of the cadaver one meter apart. As you do this you should hear the noise caused by the tearing of the sacroiliac ligaments.' "

"I can hardly wait," is a common response.

Upstairs, Steve and Jonathan are waiting to give their presentation on the abdominal cavity. Jonathan has trimmed out the abdomen neatly; Steve's tray of guts is carefully prepared. They are explaining structures to the other team members, Lisa, Jocelyne, and Cliff. They are doing such a good job that other students are gathering around as well. Steve and Jonathan are running through terms, showing muscles, nerves, arteries, and veins, as they go: "Right gastric epiploic artery"; "This can anastomose to the rectal artery"; "And here we have the lumber plexus, which consists of the following nerves. . . ." It sounds like they really know their material. They are eager to give their report and to get the hell out of there. Jonathan wants to buy a football and put it straight to use. He practices passing motions from time to time.

At the next table, Kathy is setting up her tray of guts from Nero. I am amazed how much smaller the heap is. "What happened?" I ask.

"I cut out all the fat; that's what's left."

"Wow. How long did it take you?"

"About twenty hours."

Jonathan and Steve are giving brief lectures to anyone passing by. One student asks, "Do you guys have the lumbar nerves worked out yet?"

"Here's the deal, my son," Jonathan intones, demonstrating. "Now particularly this one, the ilio-inguinal, is important, since it supplies the external genitalia. If you are thinking of cutting any of your nerves, don't cut this one." They laugh.

The presentations are going slower than usual today, because of the thoroughness of the lab instructor. The student society has three levels today: those who have presented and have joyously departed, those who are still to present, and those who are anxiously waiting to start the next dissection. A sign on the blackboard links the first two groups: HEY TEAM B——WE'LL BE AT JAGGERS CELEBRATING THE CONCLUSION OF ANOTHER DISSECTION. JOIN US!

"Try to look ready," Steve urges Jonathan as the instructor comes back in the room. They look eager and alert, but she goes to another table. "Ooooooh," they audibly moan. She promises to come to their table next. In the meantime, members of Team C are reading the syllabus directions for their upcoming work. Another sentence becomes a favorite. "Hey, guys, did you get a load of this on page eighty-eight?" Cliff calls out. " 'Be careful that the blade does not pop off of your scalpel handle during this operation and cut you,' " he reads out emphatically, raising his eyebrows.

"Oh, damn, that's what I was *planning* on," says David, shaking his head.

Much of the joking reflects nervousness not only about sexual organs, but also the structures of defecation and urination (medically styled as "micturition"). In Western culture these organs are not only private but taboo. Dr. English quoted a bit of doggerel in his lecture:

> *Although I've never seen 'em*
> *Everybody has a perineum*

partly for the joke but also to make the point that some medical training typically skips this area, even at "the finest schools." Emory students, he proclaimed, "should see——and certainly would *want* to see this part of the body."

The word *perineum* breaks down like this: *peri* means "around" and *neum* is for "anus," which basically means "ring" (as in "annual"). Yeats's poem "Crazy Jane and the Bishop" catches the many contradictory meanings invested in this piece of anatomy:

> *But love has pitched his mansion in*
> *The place of excrement;*
> *For nothing can be sole or whole*
> *That has not been rent.*

The last two lines may certainly be applied to the activity in the anatomy lab: the rending of the veils of the body leads to a wholeness in the minds of the students, an individual learning of singular things that will eventually help to heal patients, making them *whole, hale, healthy.* These last three words are related, by origin, to a fourth, *holy;* writers on medical matters often point out this family of terms, but our secular society doesn't much appreciate the implications of this linguistic unity.

As they wait to make their presentation, Steve and Jonathan suddenly break into a satiric version. Steve waves his scalpel over his tray of guts and pontificates: "And these are the brains, and this is the heart," convulsing the other students who are also painfully waiting to present or to cut. Jonathan takes up the theme, pointing to the kidneys, "And these are the testes; the first cold weather causes them to suck right back up to their point of origin." Everyone laughs with that wonderful laughter of grade school, intense, but not loud enough for *teacher to hear* (the instructor is listening to a presentation some fifteen feet away). Steve and Jonathan are our clowns, our tension relievers and creative subverters. There are jokes at every table, to be sure, but Team B from Table 3 contributes the most social forms of humor.

"Do you guys have a uterus?" a passerby asks Jonathan and Steve. "Yep, right here," they reply, pointing into the pelvic cavity. Jonathan asked Lisa and Jocelyne (who have arrived for their dissection) whether he or they could cut it open, even though that is not in the learning objectives; he wants to see inside. The students discuss with awe the notion of "a whole baby in there."

"What I don't see is how the shoulders ever get out," says Lisa, wiggling her shoulders. She turns to the cadaver and pokes around in the loose organs.

"Hey, where's our heart? You guys saw it on the exam, didn't you? It was one of the questions!" Evidently no one noticed this fact except Lisa— who spent hours and hours on that organ. Shortly she finds the heart in a plastic bag.

There is a wide variety of missing sexual organs in the women not only from surgery, but from individual variation. Little Old Lady appears to be missing one ovary. "You guys cut it out?" Jocelyne asks Steve. "Heavens no! Someone ate it," Jonathan replies. "No seriously, she apparently never had one on this side."

Finally Steve and Jonathan give their presentation and do well. They explain to Lisa and Jocelyne about spritzing down the guts and covering them with paper towels, then depart at high speed for laundry and football.

Lisa and Jocelyne have been peering into the lower abdomen, getting oriented to the uterus, the ovary, the uterine tube (also single in this specimen), and the peritoneum still covering the bladder. They have charted their strategy and now begin to cut. They peel back layers in the pelvic cavity, revealing the bladder, and cut down skin and fat over the pubic symphysis. No one seems to like these cuts into the "mons veneris," in the poetic phrase, or the "mount of Venus," which my father described to me (in a father-son sex talk) as "a kind of shock absorber." I feel a twinge of disappointment, seeing it unmasked as a mound of fat.

Further dissection bares the pubic symphysis, the meeting of the two pubic bones (expert examination of this joint can tell whether a woman has borne children, but none of us is equipped to read at that level). The women cut through the fibrous ligament, using a saw to cut one side of the bone. With pliers, they break out the bone, which is surprisingly soft. Perhaps this aged woman's bones are deficient in calcium: osteoporotic. Inside is a spongy, purplish marrow where astronomic numbers of red blood cells were formed.

This dissection proceeds from the inside out, by and large, although the external genitalia (of vulva and labia) are not cut apart. These structures stay together, like leaves in a bud.

Lisa and Jocelyne are ready to turn over their cadaver so that the buttocks and thighs can be skinned and stripped of fat.

"Will you give us a hand?" they ask me.

"Sure," I say, grabbing some paper towels.

I station myself at the cadaver's hips, more or less by instinct. The cadaver is awkward within the rails of the table. We turn her over by pulling her to one side, then up, then over. We put a block of wood under her forehead. Just beneath the sheet still covering the head, I can see small locks of gray hair on the back of her head, perhaps the most touching human sign I have seen yet in these remains.

The back has the flaps from the first dissection. "Did you see all this stuff?" Lisa asks me, pulling the flaps open and naming the muscles beneath. She has them down cold. She and Jocelyne make plans to cut again tomorrow to finish the dissection. They cover the body entirely.

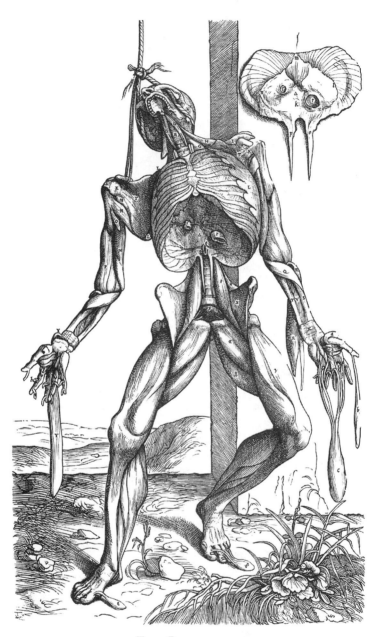

THE DIAPHRAGM

(Figure 15)

From *De fabrica,* The Seventh Plate of the Muscles, page 190.

IN THIS VERY odd view, the highly dissected body falls to the rear, so that we may look up into the rib cage, where the diaphragm usually resides. Here it has been cut away. (The lighting from the upper right shades the cavity to give an impression of depth.)

The removed diaphragm, a thin, flexible muscle, adheres (mysteriously) to the wall, looking something like a manta ray. This domed muscle separates the cavity of the lungs and heart from the cavity of the abdomen. Vesalius called it, accordingly, "the transverse septum." When it contracts, it flattens, causing the partial vacuum that draws air into the lungs for inhalation.

The diaphragm's two holes are for the vena cava (the large vein returning to the heart) and the esophagus (the food tube from mouth to stomach).

The diaphragm joins to the backside of the sternum while the two tendons that hang down (or "cura"—legs) attach to the spine. The artist has shown their corresponding white outlines on the cadaver's lumbar spine.

According to Saunders and O'Malley, Vesalius's understanding of the phrenic nerve (the motor nerve that causes the diaphragm to contract) "was one of the earliest matters in which he . . . openly announced his disagreement with Galen" (page 104).

MRS. X, J.D., GIVES BIRTH

• • •

ODAY'S LECTURE IS "Anatomy of Pregnancy and Childbirth" by Dr. English. Several students are married, but I am told that none are parents — yet. I assume that everyone in the audience is interested in sexuality and its implications. There's even a quest, a search for ultimate roots: Where did each of us originate?

"Mrs. X is a Peachtree Street lawyer who has waited to have her first child," English proceeds, telling us a story of a couple and their fetus. He uses slides to show the relevant anatomy. Mrs. X, who is not pregnant at the beginning of the story, goes to visit her OB/GYN, who performs a pelvic exam [slide] using bimanual technique (one hand in the vagina, one hand pressing on the lower abdomen). She is found to be in good health. At day fourteen of her menstrual cycle [slide of the standard Netter chart], Mr. and Mrs. X go to Atlanta's Underground, have a good dinner, a couple bottles of wine, and then return home, where they have sex [no slides]. Mrs. X has just released an ovum from her ovary through the peritoneal wall, where it floats in fluid [great slide]. The fimbriae (delicate projections at the end of the uterine tube) "are beating their little hearts out, trying to lure the egg into the tube" [slide; laughter].

"At the same time," English pauses portentously . . . then flashes up a slide of about two zillion sperm [laughter] "an *onslaught* is approaching the rendezvous. Here they are, all trying out their best lines on the ovum in the uterine tube. One smooth talker makes the connection." [The slide is an electron micrograph of a sperm penetrating—or being engulfed by—an ovum, that innermost miracle that sponsors every human being; the audience is absolutely still.] This day, however, although certainly the first day of the fertilized egg, is known as day fourteen of the pregnancy.

"I'm sorry, guys," English explains, "although sometimes women don't remember when they had sex, they always seem to remember when their last period began." Thus pregnancy dates are calculated from the beginning of the last menstrual period (or LMP). "So, crazily enough, on the day Mrs. X conceives, she is, clinically speaking, already *at two weeks.*"

When Mrs. X is late for her next period, she uses a drugstore kit to verify that she is pregnant, then makes another appointment with her OB/GYN. Since he is very popular—none but the best for this well-paid lawyer—it takes another two weeks for her to have an appointment.

In the meantime, however, her body has been changing. Her breasts have enlarged even before the time of the missed period [slide]. She has to go to the bathroom more often, because the thickening uterus is pressing on the bladder and rectum [slide]. By eight weeks, English continues, the fetus is thimble-sized [slide], and a bimanual exam shows a softening of the cervical (the neck of the uterus) and vaginal junction, another sure sign [slide]. Her blood work shows changed hormones, the most definite of all clinical signs.

At sixteen weeks, the fetus has moved up somewhat into the abdomen, giving the bladder and rectum a break [slide]. Mrs. X is thirty-five years old, having deferred childbearing until after a lengthy education and the launching of her legal career; because of her age, she elects to have amniocentesis, the drawing off of amniotic fluid for examination. (In all likelihood, some of the women students in this medical class will time their first pregnancy similarly.) Because of the possibility of genetic anomalies such as Down's syndrome in children of older women, amniocentesis is often used to verify normality in development.

English shows a slide of an ultrasound of a sixteen-week fetus. "That's my daughter," he says. [Appreciative murmurs.] Ultrasound is used to guide the narrow-gauge needle into the amniotic sac. "To the husband, this needle looks about eight feet long." Since ultrasound shows "real-time" pictures, like live TV, the action of the heart is visible, with the valves opening and closing—often a great thrill for parents to see. (The fetal heart, as everyone in the room knows from the embryology course, starts to beat on day twenty-two of gestation.) Mr. and Mrs. X choose not to know the sex of the baby. Although the test makes the sex clear, most parents choose to be surprised.

Further slides show Mrs. X's development, including a stressed look from "having the baby kicking her bladder all the time" [laughter]. Late in her pregnancy her abdominal organs are shoved to the side and, mostly, upwards, so that even her breathing is compromised. The students groan at the full-color slide, a schematic representation of the nine-month-old baby in its huge uterus, and the bowels, stomach, and diaphragm pushed away. "She doesn't want to do much besides give birth to this child," English affirms.

English describes further aspects of her prenatal care, her Lamaze classes, and the measurements of her pelvis for a determination that the baby can pass through the pelvis easily; sometimes this isn't the case, since human young have developed large heads to accommodate their large brains. Fortunately, Mrs. X comes from a family of wide pelves so the possibility of vaginal delivery looks good. Further slides describe the labor process, the various choices for anesthesia, and the descent of the baby down the birth canal, crowning into the world, turning and twisting to get the shoulders through the narrowest part of the pelvis.

"The rest of the baby comes twenty milliseconds later," English says, a fact worth knowing: this is when babies, tapering and slippery, are easily dropped—without close attention and ready hands.

The story is satisfying: we have a coherent narrative from the start to the finish of this pregnancy and the images to make it vivid. Again, the pelvis seems a place of miracles, a smithy for babies, as well as the ends of the digestive system and the seat (yes) of sexual delight. No wonder the pelvic dissection is psychologically hard to do.

WE'RE GOING TO POP HER NOW

• • •

T'S WEDNESDAY BETWEEN the regular labs, but I don't want to miss the disarticulation of the pelvis. Lisa and Jocelyne have planned to start cutting at 4:00 P.M., so I drop by about six o'clock. It takes some trial and error to get to the third floor, since the building is largely deserted, the hall lights are off, and various doors are locked. On the third floor, all doors are closed and the hallway empty, but the odor of formaldehyde is familiar, even welcome. The lights in all four labs glow through the frosted glass. I try the first door to Room 1, finding it locked, but the second door swings open.

"Pizza man!" I say, as Lisa calls out, "Howard—did you bring supper?" Not only is it truly suppertime, but an ongoing necrophagia theme refuses to die.

Four teams are at work, with only Nero and the Fatless Man covered by white plastic. Nero, however, is on everyone's mind. At the lecture this morning, Kathy came up to me and said he was found, upon being turned over, to be quite rotten. Everyone thought as much from the smell, but the students at that table had persevered in their cutting. Kathy wonders whether there will be a drastic reduction of Nero's mass, or a replacement—the two rumored solutions from previous years. I wonder whether there is ambivalence about losing him. Although he is a tough specimen to work on, the teams at Table 6 have made their peace with him; a new cadaver might require a new approach. Various students give different descriptions of the

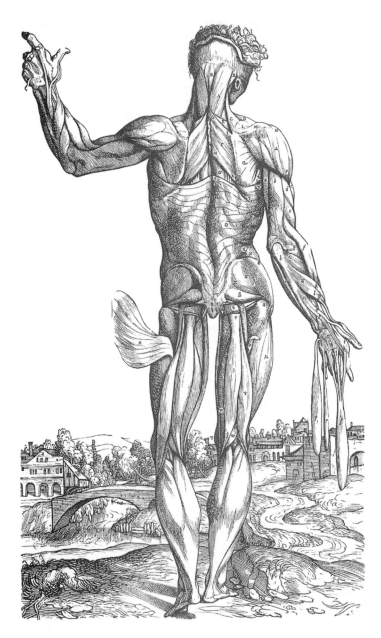

THE BUTTOCKS

(Figure 16)

From *De fabrica,* The Tenth Plate of the Muscles, page 197.

THE DISSECTION SHOWS deeper levels of the back and buttocks, where the large muscle, the gluteus maximus (labeled by Greek letter kappa—"κ"), has been turned out on the left side; on the right side, it is cut away, leaving a stub (kappa again). Underneath lie the piriformis ("β") gemelli, and obturator internus ("ε") muscles. Saunders and O'Malley believe that this is the "first illustration in the history of anatomy" to show these muscles (page 110).

Below the piriformis, the sciatic nerve sprouts out, the largest nerve cord of the body (Greek letter zeta—"ζ"), although Vesalius calls this structure a muscle. The sciatic nerve can be three-quarters of an inch in breadth. (When this nerve is irritated, the uncomfortable condition is known as sciatica.) This nerve (with both motor and sensory components) serves the skin of the foot and most of the leg, muscles of the leg and foot, and all joints of the lower limbs. "Sciatic" is a variant of *ischium,* Latin for "hip."

amount of green mold in the wide back of Nero; they all agree on the general loathsomeness of the sight and smell.

Next to the large and problematic (but covered) mass of Nero, Lisa and Jocelyne work on the buttocks and upper thighs of their cadaver in search of gluteal muscles. As they and the other teams dig deeper, the muscles emerge thick and rich. At one table the meat looks like aged raw beef.

I ask Jocelyne and Lisa about Dr. English's lecture this morning.

"I'm adopting," they reply in one voice. They particularly recall the slides showing an episiotomy (the cutting of the perineum to avoid its tearing when the baby's head passes) and the suturing of this cut. I'm sure Little Old Lady, if she had children, gave birth under different medical circumstances than do women today.

Today's dissection has much variability. Some buttocks seem to have three clear levels of the gluteus, like overlaying straps, easily separated from the sacrum and reflected back. At other tables, however, the muscle fibers appear to merge. Even the structures on the same cadaver seem to vary. At one table, one student gets the muscle layers out easily, while her partner working on the other buttock runs into trouble. Cutter 1 is having an easy time of it, for whatever reasons: the intrinsic divisions of the cadaver, dumb luck, and/or superior dissecting skills. Cutter 2, however, is having a terrible time; the fumes rise into her watering eyes and tears splatter onto her glasses. Her nose runs relentlessly. The buttock she is working on is a mess. She says something about quitting. Cutter 1, however, says, "Hey, you're doing great. You've just got to cut a little deeper and the sciatic will pop out from the piriformis. You're almost there." Cutter 2 persists and, sure enough, the structures emerge from chaos. (See Figure 16, above.)

I've seen this scenario several times: the students help each other through tough passages, when it's easy to be discouraged. Sometimes an instructor helps. One student pointed out to me a lab instructor across the room and said, "That beautiful man looked at my dissection when I was about to quit—and I mean *really* quit, the lab, the course, and maybe even the school. He said, 'This looks terrific. You've got it all here. Now just hit the books a little more to get things identified.' I'll never forget that. He really helped me up when I was down."

The students in Room 1 shuttle from table to table, learning from each other. Visitors arrive from other rooms. Dissection goes more quickly than usual tonight. There are some oddities. Some of the cadavers have a little blood in the deep areas of the pelvis—not much, but enough to notice. At Rose's table, Dave (Laird) and Chris are at work on the pelvis. They show me her ureter, which has not one but two tubes. "A bifid ureter, in about one percent of the population," Dave explains.

"We're going to pop her now," they announce to me, to the room, to themselves. This is the part of the dissection everyone has been dreading, the disarticulation of the pelvis by pulling the legs apart.

But they don't. Instead they wander down to Quasi's table to chat with Margaret and Jim, who are still picking fat from the buttocks.

At Table 2, I ask whether the cadaver has a name.

"Fred."

"Fred? How'd you get that?"

"It's for a person I didn't care too much for," the cutter says, slashing away at the buttock.

After their break, Dave and Chris come back to Rose.

"Well, I guess we gotta do it." They turn her over with care, placing a wooden block under her head. They move the books and the book stand from the foot of the table and grab her legs. They pull.

"This is terrible," one says.

"I hate this," says the other.

Everyone in the room stops work to watch this bizarre sight. The men pull the legs apart, the vulva twists and opens, and, as promised by the text, there is a deep, torturous, tearing noise. With the pubic bone already cut, the femurs (thigh bones) act like levers, pulling the pelvic bones loose from the sacral vertebrae. Some skin tears in the perineum.

"Oh God," says another cutter, watching intently, "That's awful." All the students watch, knowing they'll be doing this soon, either tonight or in tomorrow's lab.

This disarticulation of the pelvis is difficult for everyone. It is about as close to "rending a person asunder" as we are ever likely to get. To pull the legs far apart, by brute force, seems different from using a scalpel to slice the muscle. It is a grappling, a wrestling hold gone wild, something a few steps past "blunt dissection." The phrase "to pop her" is an understatement, a linguistic bandage trying to make light of the enormity of this brutal act. "Popping" a live person would certainly be in the realm of torture or rape. From the anatomical perspective, however, popping a cadaver is but one more physical maneuver in the dissection and inspection of the body, a dramatic and forceful maneuver to be sure, but perhaps not different in kind from every other anatomical action. I imagine that disarticulating the pelvis, as it occurs at the other tables, will become less dramatic, less troubling, as the students become used to it.

The opening of the vulva suggests, once again, a kind of birth, not of a baby to be sure, but of the knowledge and attitudes that form physicians. It also suggests, for the students, a loss of innocence, and a gain (or gift) of experience.

PALPATING THE LIVING
SCAPULA OF MISS Y

. . .

TODAY'S LECTURE IS on the shoulder and the hip joints. For illustration Dr. Larry Rizzolo has the usual slides, but he also uses bare human bones, his own body, and—best of all—our bodies.

"Stand up," he says halfway through the lecture, "and palpate [feel] your clavicle running from the joint at the sternum out to the acromion," the bony prominence at the top of the shoulder. We palpate our collarbones.

"Raise your hand to the side, without striking your neighbor," he continues. We chuckle and I look carefully, glad to have the opportunity to look at my neighbor on my right: I already know it is Miss Y, an image of beauty for at least some M-1 men. By chance, I am sitting one row down from the instructors' back row today. Miss Y, arriving just as lecture began, joined me. She usually sits across the aisle, farther down, with her beacon of long brown hair.

So we raise our arms without striking our neighbors, and with our other hand on top of the shoulder; thus we can verify that the arm will raise ten or fifteen degrees with its socket still. As the arm goes higher, the whole socket begins to rise as well, allowing us to put the arm directly overhead. By contrast, the hip joint will not allow such extension to the side: it is built more for stability and, of course, for bearing weight.

"Now turn to the right," Dr. Rizzolo says, "and put your right hand on the left scapula of your neighbor." I pivot to the right, while Miss Y's back,

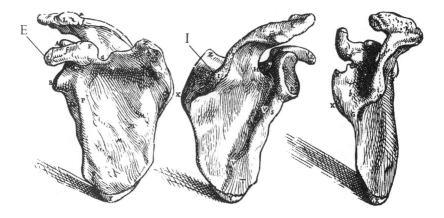

The Scapula: Three Views

(Figure 17)

From *De fabrica*, page 94.

THE LEFT VIEW is from the front of the body, so that the coracoid (crow-shaped) prominence ("E" to "F") is toward us; this prominence can be felt in the upper chest near the head of the humerus, just below the collarbone. One of the heads of the biceps originates here, and you can feel that, too, with some luck, if you flex your arm while palpating the same spot.

Scapula, in Greek, means "spade," presumably because of the shovel-like shape of the bone.

The middle view is from the rear; the spine ("I") can readily be felt on a person's back.

The right view is from the side, as if looking from the shoulder joint inwards. The four muscles that hold the humerus to both sides of the scapula are known as the rotator cuff. Baseball pitchers and orchestral conductors often tear these muscles, sometimes requiring surgical repair.

petite and trim, rotates toward me. Her hand reaches for the gross, brute back of the man ahead of her. I extend my hand to her back, gently pushing aside her thick, lustrous hair.

"Get oriented on the scapula, now, palpate the spinous ridge, running horizontally," Rizzolo exhorts us. My fingers trace along Miss Y's blouse and probe along her spinous ridge. A man would have heavier musculature: a woman's back seems open, defenseless. As Rizzolo leads us through a series of discoveries—left arm still, raised, in movement—the genius of the scapula becomes clear: it is an unusually mobile bone, adjusting to make the shoulder girdle flexible and still strong. Baseball pitchers and orchestra conductors both must take care of the four muscles (the rotator cuff) that hold the upper arm into the scapula; one exercise is to stir an enormous container of uncooked rice with the entire arm. My distraction with Miss Y's beauty gives way to anatomical insight; this back is not simply *her* back: it is a human back. I think of another emotional evolution the students are experiencing, as disgust at the cadavers yields to anatomical insight.

Dr. Rizzolo also leads us through the terminology for joint movement (abduction, adduction, extension, flexion, rotation). He explains how muscles attach to bones. Our femur (thigh bone), for example, is not simply a straight pipe, but it has curves (for strength), and outcroppings (for the attachments of tendons).

"Anatomists, being what they are, have given names to all these things, but for our purposes you don't need to know them." Just as we suspected! Anatomy is an intensely verbal discipline, as well as physical, and diagrammatic. At another point in his lecture, he mentions that the anatomical term for hip socket is acetabulum, which means "wine cup." I think of vinegar as well, since acetic acid could have the same root: the words *wine, vine, vin aigre* are all related. (According to Swinburne, the lubricious Empress Faustina, worthy symbol of Roman decadence, had a wineglass made in the shape of her breast.)

On a car trip the next day I discuss this linguistic puzzle with my colleagues, one of whom, Bob Detweiler, thinks of the *memento mori* of the Middle Ages, the empty skull kept on the writing desk to remind us that we all must die. Some of these skulls were even used as cups. (Some modern-day bars use ceramic mugs shaped like skulls for rum drinks.) My other colleague, Bill Rogers, tells a story of an Asian pilgrim who took refuge in a cave at night, awoke in the dark, and drank from what he took to be a stone. At dawn, he saw—to his horror—it was a skull into which cave water had dripped. Repulsed, he continued his pilgrimage, coming to realize that nothing inherent in the skull or water was disgusting, that the perception of the objects as repulsive was only in his own mind. Accordingly, he abandoned his trip—which was to gain enlightenment at some distant location—and started home. The enlightenment unexpectedly had come already. (Another version of this story is in Yukio Mishima's novel *Spring Snow.*)

And so it is with many of our concepts about the human body. My view of Miss Y is largely a projection of various curious dynamics of the male psyche. At another extreme of corporeal meanings are the cadavers upstairs, which society tells us are disgusting and vile. There are probably some good historical reasons for this aversion, including the avoidance of contamination and sickness. Once those risks have been greatly (or totally) diminished, once we allow our eyes to see sights that are uncommon and subversive of our usual images of health and beauty, the cadaver lying before us no longer is inherently grotesque or macabre. The cadavers, we might say, function as Rorschach tests or even mirrors of our values—values that can be changed. It puzzles me that attributed values can be very different from the symbol of them and still very powerful. I remember that my mother offered to me a beautiful pair of deerskin slippers my father wore during his final illness. I refused them, because they were, for me, sad; kneeling beside his bed many times, I had helped him put them on and take them off as he got out of bed to go a few difficult yards to the bathroom, then returned to his bed.

Upstairs, the difficult dissection of the pelvic area continues. Lisa and Jocelyne uncover their cadaver and get to work. "I'm ready to go," Lisa says, twirling her charcoal-impregnated mask on her fingers. She says that contact lenses afford more protection for the eye than do eyeglasses (despite the warning of the syllabus about possible absorption of fumes). At Table 6, the corpse remains wrapped up; there is a rumor that Nero has already been re-placed.

"You should have seen his back, man. It was all green . . . molding away," one student tells me. Others say, "Yeah, I bet that's the new one. The room smells better already!" And they get to work. (When I visit all the rooms later on, I find the Team C of Table 6 cutting in another room on another specimen. According to them, Nero is still there.)

As I think about this problem, it seems to me that the mold is an in-tensification of Nero's natural evolution in nature. The formaldehyde (like any kitchen refrigerator) retards this process, but the remains of Nero are, in a sense, "just doing their job" in their decay.

At one table, one cutter accidentally flips a small piece of the cadaver into the face of the other cutter.

"Hey, not in my face!"

"Sorry." That scrap, too, is part of the eventual disintegration of all bodies.

I feel another loosening up today among the students; there is relief from the dread of this dissection and a new confidence in facing and dealing with the job. The students have finally put their hands and minds to genitals, anus, and pelvic musculature. Now they are just working out the details.

Jokes and stories about these taboo areas are now possible, especially at one table where two men cut and others watch. They discuss various ob-jects that have been found in the rectums and vaginas of patients coming to emergency rooms. I mention a favorite slide of a radiologist I know that re-veals an entire vibrator in the sigmoid colon. The bullet-shaped cylinder shows up clearly on X ray, although the two batteries and a spiral spring con-trast best, in clear bright white. We try to imagine the plight of the patient explaining this oddity to medical personnel.

One student recalls a classmate from high school who was in the act of sitting down, naked, in the locker room. Another student (clearly a great wit) placed a pen upright on the bench beneath the bare, descending but-tocks.

"A perfect shot—went right up," he narrates.

"Ouch!" the listeners concur, giving a shiver.

"So he had to go to the hospital, where he got an enema. They got the pen out without too much difficulty, but the cap got loose and was harder to retrieve."

The students chuckle, but I can sense that they are thinking, too. This anecdote is in the genre of high-school and college wise-guy stories and medical tales told for shock value; as the students progress toward becoming doctors, however, they will hear such stories more and more as scenarios for their own actions as caregivers. Eventually they'll be in the emergency room ready to hear all kinds of bizarre tales, to which they will need to respond professionally.

By repeated and progressive contact with the cadavers, the students shape their attitudes toward subjects our society views as extreme, disgusting, and, therefore, taboo. In the emergency room I have seen nurses and physicians calmly speaking with persons covered with blood, persons who have been shot, stabbed, or beaten, persons who have traumatically lost a body part, a hand, for example. Not only do these medical personnel need to stay calm in order to do their jobs, but, in this calm or equanimity (Osler's term), they are able to help stabilize the patient emotionally, a kind of healing that can be seen not only in the patient's appearance but also in vital signs, as respirations, heart rate, and blood pressure drop back toward normal levels. I remember a nurse speaking with a distraught mother who came to the emergency room to see her daughter who had just been in a car wreck. "What your daughter needs to see right now is a very together mom. I understand that you are very concerned now, but your child is doing well and we are doing everything we can for her. You can help us by being calm yourself."

NO DESECRATION

• • •

T TABLE 2 Stephen is at work on Fred, whose penis has been sliced all the way through, like a cucumber. I look twice, never having seen a penis without its elegant end, the fruit-shaped glans; *glans* means "acorn" in Greek.

"Hey, what happened here!" I foolishly ask, knowing full well that the dissection calls for this cut.

"Not me!" Stephen avows. "I couldn't. I had Jenifer do it." Stephen and I produce little ritual laughs. The decapitated organ now looks like a little blunt sausage. If you look directly at the severed end, you can clearly see the three compartments of tissue that make up the penis, as well as the urethra, and the main blood vessels—just like, for once, the picture.

"Well, I hope it was well used in life," I mutter.

"If it wasn't, it is too late now," Stephen says.

The other cutter today is Karl, the gregarious man I remember from the heart dissection. He shows me what he has found in the perineum of Fatless Man, the muscles and ligaments, the nerves and blood vessels. While his thorax had virtually no fat, his buttocks actually do.

Karl says, "We didn't have any testes to work with here. He died of prostatic cancer, and we assume they were removed." The cadaver's legs are very thin, probably from being bedridden. There is a pressure sore (decubitus) on his hip. "And look at his legs; they're just wasted away." Sure enough, the muscle bulk of his thighs and calves is less than that of any other cadaver in the room: spindly white stalks.

"He had a really tough time at the end, it looks like," Karl says with sympathy.

Back over at Stephen's table, I look at Fred's legs. (Cadavers are left more and more bare during labs as the semester advances.) These legs are muscular and tanned; you can see a distinct line at the ankle where socks kept the skin white. "What killed Fred?" I ask.

"MI," he says (myocardial infarction, or heart attack). "We found a big bruise on his shoulder. We think that he fell." This puzzle evidently interests Karl; he comes over from his table. The two men examine the side of the cadaver's jaw, where another small wound is evident. Karl strokes the bristly ill-shaven face with his gloved hand, feeling the swelling beneath the skin. A small patch appears to have been shaven, in preparation for sewing the split skin, but we can find no punctures for sutures.

"That's strange—get him all prepped, but not sutured," Karl says.

"Maybe that's when he died," Stephen says softly.

We are all quiet a moment, aware of the enormity of this man's rapid passage from robust health to death.

Karl returns to his table, but the conversation continues.

"You know," Stephen says, "I'm so glad we don't have any desecration up here."

"Yeah, me too," Karl says.

"You hear stories . . . about other schools, where people put cigarettes in corpses, put stuff up the nose. . . ."

"Do you think that's true?"

"Yeah. It's so tacky."

(I've heard some nasty tales, some from earlier decades. A woman student, for example, was the only woman in her med school class. One day, upon undraping her cadaver, she found a cut-off penis shoved into its vagina. She survived such harassment to become a successful physician.)

Stephen's word, *desecration,* is apt, since it literally means the loss of the sacred. He is separating in his mind the disrespectful gestures from the respectful or even sacralizing ones, so that inserting cigarettes in corpses is bad, but severing the glans penis is acceptable, even an act of anatomical tribute.

On the way out, I pass by the other two rooms. At one, two women are cutting. One of them has colored the black-and-white drawings of the syllabus with colored pencils, in beautiful patterns.

"That's the way I learn it best," she says.

"Too bad the cadavers aren't similarly colored," her teammate says. But the women have created their own coloring system within the pelvis, labeling structures with strands of thread of different colors, even using a pin with a round, pink head for a structure too delicate for further dissection.

"She had lots of adhesion here following a hysterectomy. We had no uterus, no ovaries, no tubes. Just lots of scar tissue. We had a hard time separating anything," they say.

I have heard a variety of student comments about how they learn best individually: "Unless I can feel it, I can't really remember it very well"; "I've got to get it all clear from the text first"; "I've got to see it first, then go read the description." Perhaps in these various epistemologies lie some of the seeds of their future medical specialties. Some of the students dissect so quickly and cleanly that their classmates recognize their talent and the possibility that they may become surgeons. Other students who delight in all of the functions and interworkings of the thorax might be candidates for internal medicine. Students who like the interplay between models and the body might be headed for radiology and the newer imaging technologies, such as magnetic resonance imaging (MRI).

In the next room, David and Adam are cutting away at Table 17.

"How's it going?" I ask. It is almost five o'clock on a beautiful autumn Friday. Outside, the air is clear and dry, and leaves are just starting to turn. They are the only ones in the room; I imagine they might be in a hurry to get out of there.

"It's going great. We're really excited. Just look at this." Eagerly, they show me all the structures they have isolated and cleaned. Theirs is the most complete dissection of this area I have yet seen. I ask them about it, and they say, "Well, the first part was pretty bad. We were afraid that we'd ruin something. And other people did, going too quickly. It was discouraging for the first several hours, but then we got down deep enough and started finding the things we should.

"When we turned him over, we found that his rectum was full of feces. So we had to wash it all out—essentially we gave him an enema. Once that was all gone, it freed up room in the pelvis, and it got a lot easier."

"Did that smell bad?" I ask. Eventually they may have to disimpact the constipated rectum of a living person (a doctor I know at home calls this condition *dumpus constrictus*)—one of the least favorite of all physicians' (or nurses') duties.

"Not really. We think that stuff got embalmed too."

Karl has sympathy for his cadaver; Stephen is glad that no desecration comes to his cadaver; David and Adam have given an enema to their cadaver and become "excited" by the structures around the anus. Did such students have similar feelings as they worked on my father's body? What did the early anatomists feel when they stole cadavers from graveyards? Were these feelings different when they started to dissect? Is the cadaver sacred in any sense, or is it simply remains of protein and bone? The societies I know anything about all prize the remains of their dead; some even keep ancestors' bones in their homes. Our society doesn't worship the dead so overtly, but we have strong values about them, the disposition of their bodies, the legal responsibility of persons who caused death, and the like. It seems to me that any sacredness of a dead body is a value attributed not only by the society, but by the immediate observer. The students' attitudes have been evolving over the course, and now they have a working relationship with their cadavers, which includes a kind of loyalty to and honoring of the cadaver. Whether this is religious in any strict sense is debatable, I suppose, but it is certainly the kind of attitude I would have wished for my father as he lay on the stainless-steel table. Even formulating this thought is healing to me twenty-five years after his death. Our family did not experience the ritual of burial; we did not receive ashes back from the medical school. While not an enthusiastic partisan for such rituals, I have wondered whether they would have helped our grief and mourning. Instead, I find myself in the anatomy lab, assessing how my father's body may have fared. So far, I am comforted.

PELVISTON AND BEYOND

. . .

LISA AND I leave the lecture at the same time, but she beats me to the table. She's going over her notes: she and Jocelyne must give their presentation today.

"About ready?" I ask.

"Yes," Lisa says, "but we've got Dr. English!" Apparently he has the reputation for being the toughest instructor.

"Everyone says he's strict with the time," Jocelyne says.

"It's a good thing I lived in New York last year," says Lisa. "I can talk real fast now."

The room, in general, is tense, with the Team Cs worrying about their presentations, perhaps the most demanding of the semester so far. I ask Jim (Table 5) if he thinks the twenty-hour estimate (in the syllabus) for dissecting the pelvis is about right.

"That sounds a little low to me," he says. "Let's see. . . ." And he starts to add up the blocks of time he and Margaret have put in, almost every day, since last Thursday. "I'd say more like thirty hours," he concludes.

As the students practice their presentations, they turn the bodies over. I hear a student say, "These bodies have been flipped several times." This new verb "flip" suggests more ease with the turning. We are now just about halfway through the course; I think of the contrast with the first lab day when turning the corpse seemed a monumental feat. Of the six cadavers in this room, three heads are now bare, all for the first time. This is the second cycle for Team C, meaning that all of the 112 med students have now done two dissections. They are moving from levels of anatomical innocence to anatomical experience.

At Table 2 (which will present first), Stephen and Jenifer work out a scheme so that the other team members can turn the body over when Jenifer takes the instructor to the articulated skeleton: a sort of cadaveric choreography that allows demonstration of features on both sides of the body, but without wasting time within their precious ten minutes.

As I wait by the sinks, I fall into conversation with David (Team A) and the cutters of Nero. Despite all rumors, Nero is still here, freshly scrubbed down to remove his green mold. Not a trace remains. Several students ask about his condition, take a look, and pronounce him vastly improved.

Amidst this chatter David suddenly says, "You know, this cutting into bodies really leads me to see them as miraculous." He doesn't elaborate the point, but I think I know what he means: our bodies are engineering marvels, packed with nerves, arteries, muscles, bones, lymphatic ducts, all fitting together compactly, all powered by electricity, electrolytes, oxygen, and ATP in a dynamic system, ever nourishing and repairing themselves, day and night, adaptable to many climates and weathers, all functioning in families, societies, and environments—yes, miraculous.

Jim Cooper, the embalmer, stops by to check on the corpses. I ask him about his work, and he tells me that he has embalmed two corpses today. It turns out he prepares about 200 bodies a year for this university. I ask why some cadavers have incisions at the foot and ankle, others not.

"It depends whether I need to get fluid into the lower extremity, and that depends on how good the circulation system was at death," Jim says. "Circulatory illnesses pose problems for me, also kidney disease, which leaves a lot of ammonia in the body." (I learn later that ammonia is a product of tissues breaking down and remember this from the sharp smell of fish kept too long before cooking.) I am fascinated by his knowledge and how different his perspective is from mine. He sees the body as, among other things, a mobile biochemistry lab; I fled biochemistry years ago for the comfort of images, stories, and interpretations. I ask whether I can observe an embalming, and we set about figuring ways for him to contact me, since such a job occurs only when someone dies—and that can't be scheduled.

Lisa and Jocelyne are presenting, their heads bent over the pelvic cavity, along with that of Dr. English. They seem to be doing fine and finish before Dr. English's stopwatch signals *Time!* Their marks are good; others congratulate them, and they prepare to leave with smiles on their faces. I ask Lisa whether she is going to have some free time now. "Nope. Gotta hit the physiology. Lots to do there."

The last presentation today is at Table 1, where Dave and Chris have worked up a little spiel to entertain Dr. English. They were the guys who used the .22 bullet in their earlier presentation, believing that the later teams presenting should have some extra pizzazz. (Ironically, I later learn, the lecturers have a similar theory about the students, that they tend to lose interest about thirty to forty minutes into the lecture, which is, therefore, the occasion for a "wake-up slide," usually something humorous or bizarre.) Accordingly, Dave and Chris present the lower abdominal basin as "the little community of Pelviston, in the United States of Anatomy, which has recently been ravaged by Hurricancer Hugo," a reference to the September hurricane that struck the South Carolina coast. Their account continues to describe the damaged systems of this place, the plumbing (arteries and veins), the telephones (nerves), and so on. It is simultaneously ingenious and cheerfully foolish. Dr. English smiles and grimaces throughout, calling the presentation, at its conclusion, "Very entertaining . . . but so many bad puns!"

Team A returns again, ever more at home in the anatomy lab. Cliff points to the mouth of Little Old Lady and says conversationally, "She didn't have any teeth left." Her eyes are shut, mere slits. Her skin is drawn over her face. I begin to wonder whether I should even use the word *her.* Yet the body's not just an *it,* either: our language is not adequate.

Even while some of the Team C pairs are finishing up with presentations, the Team As begin to work at the tables that are ready. Today's dissection is of the shoulder and hip, parallel joints and limbs, which the students feel will be relatively easy. Indeed, work goes quickly, a good thing; this is a "quick turnaround," and they must present in two days (instead of the usual week's interval). But these joints are much easier than the pelvis— mechanically, emotionally, and anatomically. There are a limited number of objectives to be met, and the structures are much more accessible.

They start to skin back the shoulders, Cliff on one side, David on the other; this is a practical arrangement, since David is left-handed, Cliff right-handed. Little Old Lady has a lot of fat on her shoulders and upper arms, especially over her triceps (the back of the upper arm, an area American women worry about, pinch, and cover up with long sleeves). At the next table, Nero has immense muscles, easily peeled back, that look like rich steaks. At the other neighboring table, Fred has very little fat and hard, compact muscles—these also are relatively easy to dissect. Little Old Lady, it appears, is the trickiest of these three. On the other side of the room, the three cadavers who died of chronic disease have their own oddities, but I do not visit them today.

There's an easy mood to this lab session; students talk between the tables. Jonathan, having brought his football, stops by and invites us to play in the park Saturday afternoon. The jokes are gentle today. Mei hides Cliff's stool when he goes to consult a text. The contrast of this lab with the first is remarkable, when students making the first cut were nervous about their techniques, nervous about the cadavers, and, generally, strangers in this strange land.

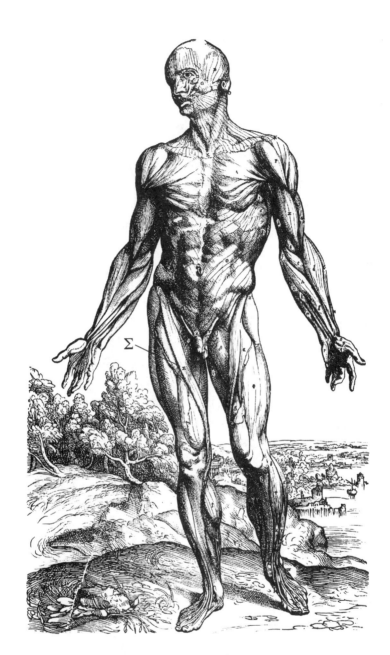

Σ

THE SARTORIUS MUSCLE

(Figure 18)

From *De fabrica*, The Third Plate of the Muscles, page 178.

THE SARTORIUS MUSCLE (marked on the figure's right thigh with the Greek letter epsilon—"ε"), is clearly shown. This is the longest muscle of the body, originating from the anterior superior iliac spine (of the pelvis), crossing the thigh obliquely, then becoming a tendon, which courses along the inside of the knee and inserts onto the upper and inner aspect of the shinbone (tibia). It is a rare "two-joint" muscle; most muscles open or close only one joint.

IS ANATOMY A DEAD FIELD?

• • •

HE LECTURE TODAY is on the thighs and knees. Jim Wilson leads us through the bones, muscles, nerves, arteries, veins, and lymphatics—the usual drill. Some words appeal to me particularly: The "hamstrings" on the back of the leg are so named because of the slaughterhouse practice of hanging up the hams of the pigs by these strong muscles and tendons. The students seem to like this fact too, giving a chuckle—while sitting on their own hamstrings.

Later, during the discussion of the knee, he invites us to feel the medial head of the tibia (the knob on the inner, lower part of the knee). "Don't press too hard; if you get it right, you can 'roll' the peroneal nerve." I press and probe without success, then pull up my pant leg and try again. Sure enough, there's the little fellow, about the thickness of a carpet thread, coursing along to supply the lower limb.

After the lecture, I ask Larry Rizzolo, who is sitting next to me, whether this class is like kindergarten for him. I have heard some of the instructors chatting about neurotransmitters, impedances, and other arcana above the level of this course. It's all new to me, something like French 101, while the professors appear to be talking about Rabelais and Proust.

"Well, some things I know well, but I need to review a lot, since we specialize so much," he says. Larry's a cell biologist, concentrating on the cellular, even molecular, level. Much of his work is with microscopes, DNA probes, and the like. "To tell you the truth, anatomy is pretty much a dead field."

"A *dead* field?" Surely he's joking. I think of the obituaries I wrote one summer for a newspaper. I learned that funeral homes participated in "stiff competition," that people "were dying to get into the obits," that my stories needed to be written "on *dead*lines."

"There are no new muscles to discover," he states. This field, in all its Renaissance grandeur, doesn't have anywhere new to go. Instead, anatomy has evolved from the "gross" level to the cellular and even molecular levels of, for example, biochemical physiology.

I'm amazed, given the immediacy and specificity in the labs upstairs, but I can see what he means. A course in gross anatomy, Rizzolo continues, is mostly "a finding-and-naming course," so that the students are oriented in basic structures and—perhaps even more importantly—basic methods of understanding: muscles and joints, blood and nerve supply, how larger and smaller structures fit together. Most of us outsiders consider the body as a black box. Pour in food and hope you'll have energy!

"They'll forget a lot of this course by their third year, when they start seeing patients in the rotations. What we hope they won't forget, however, are the methods for learning anatomy, since they'll have to learn a lot of it in greater detail for particular areas of the body." I take it he means refreshing their knowledge through texts as well as deepening their reasoning about body parts, especially those in living patients.

At one point, he says, a leading medical school thought that students forgot so much by the third year that they experimented with dropping freshman anatomy entirely, figuring it would be more efficient (and much cheaper) just to teach it all in the third year. In two more years, however—when that particular freshman class reached the hospital rotations—it became clear that the students learned less rapidly than students with a good background in anatomy. Accordingly, the freshman course was reinstated.

"We consider ourselves teachers of method. We want students to be able to solve problems, to answer for themselves the questions they raise," Rizzolo says. "Near the end of the course we get a lot fewer questions in the labs because they know how to answer them by themselves. They also know we won't just give them the answers anyway, but lead them through a Socratic path toward the answer."

Still thinking about the lecture, I ask him about the sartorius muscle, the diagonal muscle stretching from the pelvis (the anterior iliac spine) down to the inside of the knees (a tibial attachment—making it a two-joint muscle; most are one-joint). It is named for tailors (sartors), but I've never been clear why—something about how they sit, I've heard. (See Figure 18 above.)

"Well, let's see," Larry says, modeling his usual approach. "Its origin is up here"—he pokes his hip—"and the insertion is down here"—he touches his leg just below the inside of the knee. "So the axis of motion must be like this"—he raises his knee up and out. "If you contract both these muscles, you've pulled your knees apart, all ready to sit on the floor cross-legged and do some sewing." That's it, tailor fashion, or "Indian style." To me, the demonstration is the *living* anatomy, in the actual bones and muscles, as well as in this moment of teaching.

It seems to me there are two levels of anatomy: the graduate-school research model, which has evolved in areas of specialization that need new names, making anatomy "a dead field," but also undergraduate and medical models, for which anatomy is a whole new way of looking at things, particularly in a culture that has very strange notions about the body. We abuse our bodies through diet and stress; we are afraid of body smells (remember vaginal sprays?) and human excreta; we assume ideal body configurations as a norm, especially for women, so that many women feel their thighs are too heavy; we attempt to hide death. Generally speaking, the lay public is fairly illiterate about the human body, ignorant of the structures within each of us, and, therefore, prey for any pharmaceutical company that advertises some nostrum to cure our ills through chemistry. As one doctor expressed it to me, "No matter how smart or well educated, most Americans have only a primitive understanding of how their bodies work."

A SERIOUS, MAJOR-LEAGUE
SOMETHING OR OTHER
• • •

I
T'S A HAPPY day: The fall weather is beautiful, the pelvis is past, and the upcoming arm dissection is considered easy. It's exactly halfway through all the anatomy labs, but Team A, reporting today, actually breaks the midpoint, giving the third presentation of five: *Only two more dissections!* they boast. Some are now hosting prospective students, visiting from their undergraduate campuses, all stiffly dressed in Good Clothes. This new medical underclass in the making assures the current M-1s that they will no longer be freshmen but will next summer become exalted M-2s!

The lecturer today, Dr. Steven Wolf, says that the material he has to present (on bones and joints) "isn't, frankly, terribly interesting," but that he'll do his best to spark things up with a videotape of arthroscopic surgery. The students chuckle at his candor.

So Wolf dutifully tells us about bones (living tissue), and joints (fibrous, cartilaginous, synovial), and gives us new vocabulary (fossa, sulcus, foramen, etc.). Then he shows the tape of the inside of the knee, as seen through the arthroscope—a thin tube with tiny surgical devices as well as fiberoptic filament that lights and videotapes the area. Thus the surgeon can watch the operation on a nearby TV screen intently. "Remember, this is fifty times the size of the actual interior," Wolf says, as we watch a slender but visually enormous instrument trim a torn meniscus, while the fragments rush away in a stream of saline solution.

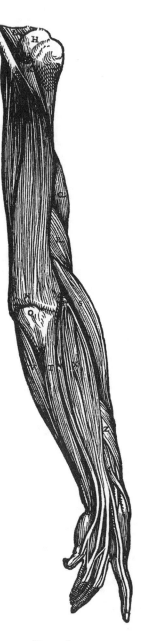

THE ARM

(Figure 19)

From *De fabrica*, page 219.

THIS RIGHT ARM has been dissected from the shoulder. "H" represents the head of the humerus, a ball that fits into the approximate socket of the scapula and the collarbone or clavicle (literally "little key," the strut between sternum and arm). It's not unusual for a shoulder to "separate," or dislocate, because it is unstable compared to the hip.

Just out of sight in this woodcut, behind the elbow, courses the ulnar nerve, between the heads of the ulnar bone ("O") in the forearm and the inner condyle (or "knuckle") of the humerus; it tingles when bumped: the funny bone.

According to Saunders and O'Malley, there was much confusion among the ancients about nerves, tendons, and muscles: "He's got some *nerve*," we still say of a forceful person. Vesalius began to see distinct differences between the two, as shown in the forearm of this illustration. Particularly at the wrist, we see how tendons for extending the fingers grow out of the muscles.

Coming around the podium to speak informally, Wolf ends his talk with a joke: "A woman recovering from hip surgery is ready to go home. The Big Doctor arrives with his entourage in tow. The lady asks whether she can resume sexual relations at home. The Big Doctor says, Well, if sex were *play,* I'd say yes, but since we all know it's *work,* I'll have to give the order no."

"Outside the woman's room, Big Doctor quizzes the entourage on the lady's medical status and on his wise advice." (And here Wolf says, "We're all aware of pecking orders in the medical world, aren't we?" The students vigorously nod their heads in agreement.)

"The chief resident—finishing his training, and shortly looking for a job—says, 'Oh yes, you are *so* right. Sex is one hundred percent work. Everyone knows that.' The first-year resident, hoping to be impressive, says, 'But I've recently read an article in the *New England Journal of Medicine* that more accurately sets parameters of eighty percent work, twenty percent play.'

"Next, the fourth-year med student says, 'Well, I'd say fifty-fifty. As a matter of fact, there was an article in *JAMA* with similar figures.'

" 'And in your opinion?' Big Doctor asks the first-year med student.

" 'I'd say one hundred percent play.'

" 'All *play,* you say. Really! What's your proof? Any citations?'

" 'Nope. I just know if there was any *work* involved, I'd be doing *yours!* ' "

The students laugh uproariously. For them it's a recognition of the ranking in the profession that finds them currently on the bottom: during their hospital rotations in their third and fourth years, they'll be doing a lot of "scut work" for residents or attending physicians, drawing blood, arranging tests, doing workups. (There is even a book called *The Effective Scutboy: The Principles and Practice of Scut,* 1988.) Furthermore, the Freudian attack on the professor is delightful, particularly the Oedipal suggestion of sexually taking his wife. That Wolf should break the frame of his lecture to tell his joke seems an avuncular act, acknowledging the folk wisdom of the medical subculture.

Upstairs, Cliff and David are ready with their presentation on the shoulder and the hip. Steve, Jonathan, and Lisa stop by to observe.

"Hey, that's gorgeous. You guys tagged them really well," Jonathan says of the carefully prepared dissection with streamers of multicolored thread. Cliff and David seem quietly proud of their work.

Before long, though, it's time for them to perform. Dr. English starts the clock, and Cliff and David methodically go over the bony landmarks, the arteries, and the veins. The spectators watch respectfully, but nothing really exciting has happened yet. Suddenly David's voice assumes the dramatic urgency of a radio announcer and he cries out, "It's John Elway stepping up to the line, third and long!" As David gives the spiel of Elway's activities, Cliff pantomimes them in exaggerated slow motion. Cliff, in his white lab coat and glasses, pulls his arm back to throw, hurls the arm and ball forward, and pulls his arm back to the body—David halloos, "Just before the linebacker crashes in on the doomed quarterback!" All during this David points out with his forefinger the location of the abductors, rotators, extensors, and adductors on Cliff's shoulder.

"And the pass is good, a touchdown!" he finishes in a roar. Students at other tables stop work and watch the drama.

For the point-after-touchdown attempt, Cliff takes up the description, while David slowly goes through a kicking motion. "Since he's a soccer-style kicker, the rotational muscles of the pelvis are important. The kick is up and good! The referee signals that the kick is good by raising his arms—lateral rotation and abduction!" Cliff cries out, his arms dramatically raised. The other students laugh and cheer at this brio.

At the end Dr. English says, "That was great. I liked it, and I especially appreciated the demonstration of the movements. That shows that all these structures do something and aren't just abstract entities." He goes on, "I'm blown away by your obturator internus nerve—really well displayed. In general this is a very clean dissection. Great job."

English goes on to another table while Cliff and David receive congratulations from their colleagues. They are relieved and happy. David takes off, but Cliff stays around the lab for another hour, winding down, looking into cadavers and talking with the other students—wearing his backpack all the while. Dr. English moves to the next table, Nero's, where Aravind and

Mike are wearing bright yellow gloves. Everyone notices this dramatic departure from the tan latex gloves and asks about them.

"We got tired of those damn latex things tearing all the time. Besides, no more dishpan hands for us!" The gloves are, in fact, kitchen gloves. They have written on them little phrases: *Dr. English rules* and *Dr. English kicks ass.* Dr. English, approaching their table, notices the spectacular gloves but not the writing thereon. He asks, "Do you wish to acknowledge wardrobe help?" and they get right to work. Following the presentation, however, the students specifically show Dr. English the mottoes. He seems to accept the implied notoriety.

Meanwhile, Steve and Jonathan have taken up their position at Table 3. "Okay, let's turn this thing over," Steve says, and he and Jonathan turn Little Old Lady onto her back again. They neaten up the work space, drape the legs and face, and extend the right arm for dissection of the brachial plexus (the upper arm, particularly the structures in the armpit).

"Here we go, dudes; watch this two-handed pullback!" Jonathan announces as he forcibly pulls back the skin on the upper arm with his gloved hands.

There is a new freedom for a lot of the students, as they ignore the *Dissector* and even speak disparagingly of it ("Not worth shit"). At the beginning of the course, they followed it slavishly. Now, they ask around among the tables and see the fastest way to get out what they need, which usually means cutting directly through some features. In the phrase from the theater, they consider themselves "off book," as if they know their lines by heart and can now put on the play without the text in hand.

"This is going to be a good dissection," someone says.

Jonathan finds a network of long, linking veins. "Hold it, everybody, we've got a serious, major-league something or other here!" The blood vessels and nerves running through the armpit look like a tangle of off-white strings. As you look more closely, the veins are smaller, more stringlike, while the arteries are larger and harder, more like the little tubes they are in life. The arteries have thicker and tougher layers, which keep their shape after death. The veins, however, are more slack and collapse upon themselves, like loose cotton cords. Veins are not very strong; under pressure, they can swell out, becoming varicose. One lecturer described hemorrhoids as varicose veins and asked, "Who gets these?"

"Weightlifters!" was the immediate response of the men, some of whom have experienced this problem. An instructor at my elbow added under his breath, "And jet pilots." "Huh, how's that?" I asked. The former navy fighter pilot explained: "We'd pull four Gs pretty often. The blood just pools."

Nero's is the last table for presentations in the lab today, so Kathy and Elizabeth get a late start. "Okay, you big guys, who's going to help us turn Nero over?" one of them asks. Several men drop everything to do the job, and soon Kathy and Elizabeth are cutting away. The Table 1 team has brought a radio, and it becomes my job (as nongloved) to plug it in and find a rock station. Soon the students are singing along with songs they know—and I don't.

Jonathan and Steve seem excited about hosting a prospective student. They are, provisionally at least, successful medical students anxious to pass on their hard-earned wisdom to a neophyte—a role they played one year ago. I am not surprised to learn that the student they have volunteered to help is female. Jonathan leaves to meet Ms. Prospective Medical Student, so I chat with Steve while he cuts the skin and fat away from the forearm. He tells me about a letter he and Mei wrote to a patient who appeared in the biochem class. An alcoholic with a variety of medical problems, she appeared in a "clinical correlation" format, a living example of some of the abstract principles in the course. "She got outta there so fast, none of us could thank her, and she shared a lot of heavy-duty stuff. So we just had to write her a letter to express our gratitude." I see in this the empathy that will help make Steve and Mei good physicians.

The corpse at the next table, Fred, has a big bruise on the inside of his elbow, probably representing the last attempts at the IV therapy to save him from his heart attack. This area is known as the "antecubital fossa" or the "hollow in front of the cubit," a rare use of the biblical word. Anyone who has given blood has gotten stuck there.

Jonathan comes back, annoyed that he could not find Ms. Prospective Student.

"Your turn, babe," he informs Steve, jerking his head toward the door.

"What we got here so far?" Steve fills him in on the dissection and warns him that the arm is messy, dripping fluid and liquid fat onto the floor. At all tables, one arm extends perpendicular to the body, straight off the table, while the students sit on a stool within this strange one-armed embrace. Of all the cadavers, Nero has the biggest arm. Little Old Lady's arm is slim.

I look at this thin arm sticking out into space. It had a long history, a hundred years of human activities, some of which were routine, "activities of daily living," in the phrase of the physical therapist, or ADL. Certainly she dressed herself, brushed her hair, cooked, did laundry. And what else might be part of the history of this arm? What lover(s) did she hold? What children did she help dress? Did she ride a horse? Turn the pages of a book? And it is still working, in a sense, as it teaches Steve and Jonathan its slowly revealed structures.

Jonathan surveys the arm, which is now coming apart, and dripping on the floor.

"That's okay," he says. "We'll just put down more paper towels." His attitude is matter-of-fact, but the phrase catches my attention. Halfway through the course, this strange mess is, for him, "okay," normal, natural, part of what the anatomical process is all about.

As Steve goes to try again to find Ms. Prospective, Jonathan dissects the superficial veins of the arm and cuts off big hunks of the skin, now freeing the arm from the armpit to the wrist. He must eventually shell all the fat out of the armpit so that all the connections of the nerves and vasculature become clear. His methods are neither orthodox nor prim.

Dr. Wolf sticks his head in the door, and there are some wisecracks between him and the students, especially Jonathan.

"You weren't thinking of surgery, were you?" Dr. Wolf asks Jonathan.

"Oh, definitely!" Jonathan smiles beamingly.

"I never saw any one dissect *quite like that.*"

"Whatever works," Jonathan replies, unruffled. The other students enjoy the repartee. In his clownish way, Jonathan is a symbol, a champion of their freedom.

Dr. English sticks his head in the other door. The mood is loose enough for someone to ask one of The Questions so far repressed.

"Can you get AIDS from a cadaver?"

"I don't think anyone has verified that . . . only slow viruses."

It seems that the AIDS question is central enough to take all the attention. No one asks what a slow virus is. After all, if you survive the first semester of med school, making it to Christmas, anything else can be dealt with later.

FEMORAL/EPHEMERAL

. . .

ORE ANYWHERE?" SOME twenty men in the class greet each other with this ritual phrase. We had gathered the previous Saturday afternoon in a park to play football. It was a beautiful day, sunny, cool, and dry. No one talked about med school: the game was an escape, a tribute to autumn, "Season of mist and mellow fruitfulness," in Keats's words. Upon our return to the anatomy-physiology building, evidence of the game comes along too, and the men tell each other where they are sore or bruised. I have a sore ear to report, caused by someone's enthusiastic forearm. (Jonathan later claims, with a mixture of apology and pride, that it was his.) The meaning of our game is a humanizing strand within these strange walls, and the players have a fuller sense of each other as people, not just fellow dissectors. Different medical specialties—family medicine, surgery, psychiatry—have different ways of balancing technical expertise with human compassion, or "bedside manner," as it was once phrased. In this anatomy class, the cadavers have been largely seen as scientific exhibits, but there is also now a countermovement as the students interpret clues to the past lives of the cadavers, a symbolic rehumanizing of them.

Today's weather, by contrast, is hot: oppressive and gray, packed with humidity. Although the trees are turning yellow, gold, and orange, although the leaves are starting to drop on the lawns and sidewalks, this day feels like August, and everyone complains. "I'm sweating bullets," Jonathan gripes up in the lab. The weather reports promise cool, dry air sweeping in from the northwest, but it damn sure isn't here yet.

The lecture went ten minutes over today, an unusual event. Dr. Wolf packed his time with terms, slides, and demonstrations while discussing the forearm and hand; the demonstrations were the most vivid, since each of us had exhibits "at hand" to refer to.

"Feel thyself!" Dr. Wolf exhorted. "We will have self-palpation today." [Laughter.] "Why is it that the guys always get excited?" [More laughter.]

Upstairs, the Team Bs are ready to present. Steve and Jonathan have done a careful job cleaning up the armpit and upper arm of Little Old Lady. They have placed pieces of electrician's tape to mark the strings that hang from the torso to forearm, green for nerves, red for arteries, and blue for veins.

"Nice flags, guys," a classmate says.

Apparently Steve and Jonathan feel secure about their presentation, since they aren't practicing it. I compliment them on their dissection, and Jonathan says, "Well, it took some time. It really was a mess of spaghetti, but it's pretty cool now."

When it's time for the presentation, Dr. Wolf starts his stopwatch, and Jonathan boldly declares, "Let's start with the M shape here." (The lecturer stressed this oddity, a pattern of the upper arm nerves that creates a large letter M.) "Obviously it stands for the University of Michigan, national champions." He gestures to Steve, who dramatically opens his lab coat to reveal a shirt that reads MICHIGAN: ON THE ROAD TO THE FINAL FOUR—CHAMPS.

This tribute to their alma mater accomplished, Jonathan and Steve take turns explaining the structures of the arm. They start with about eight listeners. The room is quiet, and the presentation is clear. By the time they finish, fifteen students are standing around the table, craning their necks to see the exhibit. "And that's all we'd like to talk about today," the presenters finish up.

"Why did Notre Dame beat Michigan?" is Dr. Wolf's first question. Everyone laughs.

After the discussion of the presentation, the men go out into the hall for feedback from Dr. Wolf, who comments on three or four errors in their work, but congratulates them on their overall excellence and awards them a 6. They return to Table 3, to gather their things and to fly—if the past is a guide—out of the lab. Today, however, they start explaining their work to Lisa and Jocelyne, who are there for the next dissection. Slowly and carefully, they go over all the structures again, answering questions; another two students join the group. David is there, too. He asks, "Oh Great One, show us the lymphatic system." It's a joke, but also a tribute. This Team B really knows the topic. (And the Latin root of *doctor* means "teacher.") They help their colleagues for forty-five minutes. When they do finally gather their things for departure, Steve says, "This was the most fun dissection. We really got into it!"

"This will be nothing like the last dissection we did [the dreaded pelvis]," Lisa says, while she and Jocelyne put on their new scalpel blades. "Besides, I've always been interested in legs." It turns out she watched some twenty arthroscopies last year, most of them on the knee; indeed she wrote a research paper on the topic. She and Jocelyne start right in on a thigh, cutting through the skin, pulling it back, and removing large amounts of yellow fat. Very soon they start to separate the large muscles of the upper leg. The sartorius crosses the thigh at a jaunty angle. This dissection goes very quickly at all tables, because of the relative ease in defining these body parts, and, of course, because of the students' improving skills.

When Dr. English stops by, students ask him about opening the windows for some more air; it feels oppressive in the lab today. A chalk drawing on the blackboard shows the doors to the room and the windows— marked DIRE SITUATIONS ONLY.

"There are two reasons we can't open those, not even counting the objections of the secretaries in the next building," Dr. English says. "First, the air conditioning can't work right in removing air from this room; it ends up going all over the building, and we get complaints. Second, mold spores come in and get on the cadavers." In this brief speech, he sums up several of the dilemmas of dissection: there is a taboo against seeing it, there is a taboo against smelling it, and it's hard technically to keep the cadavers in good shape, that is, to obstruct the natural forces of disintegration. (In Renaissance medical education, anatomy was scheduled for the winter term, so that the corpses would decompose more slowly.)

There is some discussion about the proper accent on the word *femoral,* which leads to a pun on the word *ephemeral.* (*Hemera* means "day" in Greek; insects are traditionally "ephemeral," dying after short lives.) The deaths of the corpses are on the students' minds today, because the embalmer has cut into the upper thigh on most of the cadavers, leaving some damage to the femoral artery, which supplies the thigh. Several students mutter complaints about this, since they fear it will look like they haven't dissected carefully. How ephemeral is the femoral area? How ephemeral are any of us? We are moving toward the time of the year when the first frost will kill all the insects that chirp and sing at night.

Dr. Wolf comes back to the lab to visit, sitting casually on a stool between two tables. He's had a busy afternoon already, first giving a seventy-minute lecture, then hearing and responding to six student presentations for another ninety minutes or so. He's glad to unwind with students and make conversation. Thus, he is now a less frightening figure than the evaluator of just an hour ago. Karl and Charlie ask Dr. Wolf about the cuts on the thigh.

"Well, that's to exsanguinate the corpse, naturally. Some embalmers inject water and run that until all the blood is out. Others start in right away with the preservatives. There's all sorts of different ways." He and the students talk frankly about where the bodies have come from, how they are handled, where they go besides this lab. It's a factual and healthy discussion; most of the cadavers come from hospitals or nursing homes where the death occurred. The legal directions for a body provide that it be delivered directly to the university, which becomes responsible for the embalming, use, and final disposition. This information was given to them at the beginning of the course, but evidently they need to hear it again now that they know their cadavers better.

"Did they know they were going to end up here?" someone asks.

"Sure, either here or for research within the department. Yes, this is what they intended and filled out papers for," Dr. Wolf replies. "We can't—and shouldn't—know more about them personally. They may have many different kinds of reasons." Some students nod their heads, glad to have this validation.

One student asks about a rumor he's heard, that there might be a pool somewhere with lots of corpses. I try to picture this bizarre image.

"Not here. We handle them individually, although there was a school that appropriated a swimming pool that could no longer be used for phys ed and floated their cadavers in that."

I try to sort out my emotions regarding my father's journey. As a child I felt awe for his size, his strength, the warmth of his body. In the year prior to his death I—that is *we*, the entire family—felt much sadness in seeing his physical abilities and his body itself deteriorate. Following brain surgery and radiation therapy, he appeared to have aged two or three decades in an accelerated leap toward senility and death. He had been an active man, swimming (which maintained his body), doing intense intellectual work (which maintained his mind). Suddenly, he had terrible losses in both body and mind. Clearly death would come—we just didn't know when. I remember worrying about how to broach the topic with him. One supper with my mother in the kitchen, I drank an entire bottle of red wine, then went back to his bedroom. I lay on the bed next to him; he could barely move.

"Dad?"

"Yeah."

"Do you know you're going to die?"

"Yeah."

"Are you . . . okay with that?"

"Yeah . . . pretty much. Yeah."

I have wished our conversation were somehow deeper, but maybe that was enough. It was the best I could do at the time, and maybe all he could do. At any rate, I felt better and hoped he did too.

A religious family, we believed his soul would gain freedom at his death, leaving the dross of the body behind. I hope he's having spiritual adventures in the beyond. William Blake, for example, hoped he would be able to converse in heaven with John Milton. I think my father would enjoy talking with no end of intellects, artists, and visionaries, including Milton, Blake, Eleanor Roosevelt, and the Beatles; I hope that is happening right now and that someday I'll join in the conversation.

Still, it was his body, uniquely his, that we saw falling apart, that we dealt with every day. I hope the arrangements of the medical school that received his body were humane and respectful.

THE FIRST INTEROSSEUS
OF A PIANIST'S HAND

• • •

I'S COLD THIS October day, unseasonably and absurdly cold. I walk to work in a windy fifty-three degrees, the high for the day. The temperature—under gray, forbidding skies—plummets all day, as cool air pours in from Canada. It is a quick change of mood, and the students wear sweaters and jeans in the lecture hall.

Today's lecturer is Dr. Foad Nahai, a plastic and reconstructive surgeon. Although he works on many areas of the body in his practice, his specialty is the hand. His lecture then is part of the pedagogy of "clinical correlation," which intends to show how knowledge of anatomy helps to heal actual living human bodies.

Dr. Nahai has us all move down to the front of the auditorium so that we can see better, he says (although it becomes apparent that he wants to see us better too). "In all probability, only a fraction of you will follow in my professional path," Dr. Nahai says, "but all of you will shake the hands of your patients, feel their pulses, and be asked by friends and neighbors about possible hand damage."

Dr. Nahai reviews the basic terminology and structures of the hand, using his own hands prominently—these hands that perform microsurgery on nerves, blood vessels, and tendons. He asks us to examine our own hands, those wonderful assemblages of twenty-six bones apiece (counting the wrist bones). The hands and feet account for over half of the bones in the body: this large number is important for strength and flexibility.

"How many of you have a palmaris longus on both hands?" he asks, and we all raise our wrist and flex our hands toward the elbow. This muscle (with the tendon linking forearm to hand) is frequently absent on one or even both sides; its presence makes little difference, since it is a weak flexor of the hand. It can be seen indirectly, by its tendon near the wrist tenting the skin like a pencil under a cloth napkin.

"Oh my God," jokes a nearby man. "I must be a mutation. I thought that I was perfect. That's what my Mommy always said!" He has no palmaris longus in one arm, but another student in front does, and Dr. Nahai congratulates her: "You've got a good one. You should come up front!" Everyone laughs. Since this muscle is not much used by human beings (although it is important to tree-hanging monkeys), it is often taken out and moved for tendon grafts. Dr. Nahai later shows us slides of severed tendons in the back of the hand which have retracted some two inches back into the wrist. A transplanted palmaris longus tendon makes the hand functional again by reconnecting the forearm muscle to the fingers. It's amazing that many of the functions of the hand are done by remote control: much musculature is in the forearm, while a series of ingenious tendons link up to the hand's bones, giving us strength and flexibility down to our fingertips.

Dr. Nahai shows a series of slides of hands, asking students to identify the injured portion and to define the loss of function. Some of these appear to be relatively simple injuries, such as minor cuts or stabs, but even a small cut can cause a finger not to work. I feel some gratitude for cuts on my hands over the years that have never done any major harm. Once I cut across the web between thumb and forefinger, good for seven stitches; fortunately the cut was not deep. I look at the pale scar now. The emergency room doctor did a nice job; I wish I could thank her. I remember that she asked how I gashed my hand. I explained that I foolishly used a butcher knife to pry coconut meat from a shell and, well, the knife slipped. "Ooogh." She shivered. "How come you can sew up hands but don't like the stories?" I asked her. "The sewing I can control," she replied, readying her hypodermic.

I see students examining their own hands, as if for the first time in a long while, tracing scars, making fists, wiggling their fingers. These hands will touch, will heal, will comfort many people over the next decades.

Other slides show more serious injuries, such as amputations of fingers; in some cases Dr. Nahai and his colleagues can replant these (or move a toe up to the hand as a replacement) in an operation lasting four to twelve hours. Unlike the bloodless bodies upstairs, these slides show bloody tissue in bright, danger-signaling scarlet. Students make the sound of "Ooooooh" for several of these, especially the lawn-mower injuries. "I do not own a lawn mower," Dr. Nahai says simply.

"As physicians, we must be aware of the enormity of disability for our patients," Dr. Nahai concludes. "To be missing fingers on both hands may make going to the men's room by yourself impossible. We must realize the human meaning of such losses and do our best to help our patients."

It is a valid and inspiring lecture. With their perfectly working hands, the students give Dr. Nahai a warm round of applause. They talk about his remarks while going upstairs and through the next few hours of dissection.

"You could hang meat in here, ha ha ha," jokes Lisa, upon entering the lab upstairs. It is in fact extremely cold. Giving off roughly 100 watts of heat apiece, the students will slowly raise the temperature of the room; the cadavers, of course, will not contribute any heat, but their temperature may fractionally rise as the room warms. Lisa and Jocelyne prepare to present the thigh.

Little Old Lady lies on her back, her right leg fully dissected. What jars the eye is the thin, frail set of muscles inside what was, apparently, a full leg: she had a good inch of fat all around, a real blanket of yellow cells. By comparison on either side, Fred and Nero have huge muscles, bulky as ropes, with very thin layers of fat. The three chronics, across the aisle, have wasted muscles, even frailer than Little Old Lady's.

I think of the signaling value of subdermal fat, especially in women. The fat on a woman's thigh is important to men, for reasons they don't generally understand, but these reasons help the human race to continue. Part of a man's job—as created through evolution—is to locate women with enough subdermal fat for pregnancy, childbirth, and the comparatively long infancy of human young. At some 3,700 calories per pound, fat is a very efficient method of storing fuel. Little Old Lady's fat was just doing its job, although her childbearing years had ended roughly five or six decades ago.

Despite the gloomy weather, it's a day of high energy inside. Students banter and josh, talk about the lecture, and make the ritual jokes about the upcoming presentations. As Lisa talks to David, she bangs her probe on his chest. She and Jocelyne have done a good job finishing up the leg; shortly they will present. Charlie tugs at my sleeve: "You've got to hear the presentation in the next room!"

I race next door, where Lisa (Drake) and Gail are presenting the thigh and knee at Table 9. They are wearing aerobics clothes under their lab coats, and the cadaver, improbably enough, is wearing a pair of Reeboks and sweatbands at the wrist. Fully twenty students are gathered around, some kneeling on stools to see better, while the women give the information within an ingenious narrative of an aerobics class: "Let's warm up and get the blood flowing!"; "Let's stretch the following important muscles!" They talk in the jovial commands of an aerobics instructor, exhorting their clearly dead participant to ever greater efforts. Even this ironic presentation suggests the former life of the cadaver, whose knees once bent, whose legs once moved. By the end of the presentation, still more students have clustered around, filling most of the room; they applaud vigorously, part of this celebrative ritual. Having given presentations, all of them know what kind of effort goes into a good one.

Back in Room 1, Lisa and Jocelyne have presented and done well. They are excited at being finished and whiz out of the room. At the board, Jim is carefully diagramming part of the leg for three students. Someone pokes me and says of him, "He's a born teacher."

The room is noisy today. The students recall slides from the hand-surgery lecture. One tells of a lawn-mower accident in his own family and the replantation of three toes on his father's foot. "And this was years ago, man." Another tells about a family boat accident and the subsequent medical treatment. The students seem energized and focused on medical topics today; they have momentum.

David and Cliff take over at Little Old Lady's table; they are assessing her hands, the subject of today's dissection. Their young, pink hands are flexible, even in the latex gloves; they hold her ancient hands, now gray and stiff. "Damn," says Cliff, "we should have tied these back somehow so that they would be nice and open to work on. Why didn't we think of that?"

"Yep . . . these will be hard to get into," says David. The books, they tell me with scorn, show entirely cooperative hands, flat as pancakes.

They cut away, skinning down the hands, picking the fat. We talk about the muscles and tendons. I remember a comment by one of the anatomy instructors: "A piano player will have a huge first interosseus muscle, from reaching with the index finger." This muscle ("between the bones") is readily felt between the thumb and forefinger; if you reach the forefinger toward the thumb, you can feel it contract and bulge. Similarly the musculature of every cadaver has been shaped by the activities he or she participated in. Even the skeleton itself selectively lays down more bone to handle the increased muscular load. In some absolute sense, every single body (living or dead) in this lab is a text, a record of a lifetime of activity, if only we could read it.

"Can we tell whether she was right- or left-handed?" I ask Cliff and David.

"Not yet, but maybe when both hands are stripped."

The chronic patients across the aisle all have muscles atrophied down to a minimum. Is it better to die used up or to die in robust health like Nero and Fred? As Tennyson put it in "Ulysses":

> How dull it is to pause, to make an end,
> To rust unburnished, not to shine in use!

When Cliff asks me to take his glasses from his face and to put them somewhere, we make some jokes about where and he says, "Well, you could put them on the cadaver." We chuckle and let it drop, but I think about these glasses and the Reeboks from the aerobics presentation as symbolic attempts to "reanimate" these cadavers, not literally, of course, but as tributes to the past humanity of these bodies, which are now pretty heavily cut up.

Another trajectory is underway, the yearly project of the Chaplain Donald Shockley to plan a Service of Reflection and Gratitude. Don has put notices in all the students' boxes and a sign-up sheet in the mail room. In just one day, all fifteen slots are filled in with names of volunteers, and a few extras have been added around the edge as well. Evidently there is considerable interest—perhaps even a hunger—to work on this project as a way of bringing closure to the cutting.

I fall into conversation with a blond man I haven't met. He says that he was sometimes angry at his cadaver early in the course ("Why do you have to have such thick skin?") but now feels guilty about such anger because, as he cuts deeper, he finds "a marvelous inner structure" in the body, for which he is "truly grateful." Later it occurs to me that while I don't know all of the 112 students, all of them know by now who I am; since I have no official role in these proceedings (certainly not any ability to give grades), I am a safe person to talk to.

Another instance of such growing sensitivity is at Table 1, the home of the ingenious framing tale for presentations, such as the cardiac gunshot and Hurricaner Hugo striking Pelviston. "Any great stories for today, guys?" I ask.

"Nope, not today. We were thinking about one with the San Francisco earthquake, but we watched the news and saw the collapsed interstate with some two hundred people reported dead . . . and we bagged it. Some things you just do not joke about. We'll do this one straight."

We talk about the horror of the event, particularly the young boy saved by rescue workers who cut through his dead mother with a chain saw and amputated one of his legs as well to rescue him. We shudder with horror. To be a physician is to commit yourself to confront such horrors and to use your skills and knowledge to do what you can to bring comfort and healing to patients.

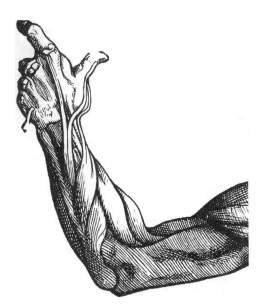

The Anatomical Snuffbox

(Figure 20)

From *De fabrica,* The Tenth Plate of the Muscles, detail, page 197.

IN THIS UPRAISED left hand, the two extensors of the thumb stand out in white. Where they join the wrist, they form the "anatomical snuffbox," which can be seen and felt on a living hand, by strongly raising and extending the thumb away from the forefinger. Snuff dippers could place morsels of tobacco here before sniffing them.

AND IN MY BRAIN

• • •

THE LECTURE TODAY might be more accurately called a demonstration: Dr. Wolf has two live persons to present to the students. I come in late and see the second patient only, a boy of about twelve who was in a car accident eight years ago. He suffered a serious head injury, which left him in a coma. After regaining consciousness, he had only limited therapy for his atrophied muscles. Dr. Wolf and others are now trying to assess his status and give him the best possible program of rehabilitation. Many of the abstractions of the past lectures suddenly come into focus as Dr. Wolf has Sam (a pseudonym) walk across the platform, swaying and lurching, according to his weak muscular groups, those that cannot "work synergistically in maintaining erect posture, balance, and locomotion," in Wolf's terminology. The act of walking even by the healthy suddenly seems forbiddingly complex: estimates suggest that over 200 muscles are used in walking, muscles in the legs and arms, of course, but also many stabilizing muscles in the torso.

"Boy, a lecture like that really helps your motivation," Doug says, upstairs. "If I ever have patients like that, I need to know the muscle groups, the innervations, and the point at which to refer to a specialist!" Another lesson comes through as well: not only does Dr. Wolf know what he is talking about structurally, but he also appears to have a close relationship with his young patient. I like the way he talks to him, touches him, and congratulates him on his progress. We hear about "heartless medical technology," and we sometimes overlook the small acts of kindness bestowed by physicians, nurses, therapists, and other medical caregivers. Dr. Wolf treats his young patient as a person with a difficult past, yet a promising future.

In the lab, all is quiet when I walk in. There are only a few students at work, and there are no presentations today. The dissection of the hand is finished at most tables, and the six white cocoons lie undisturbed. Taking advantage of a less pressing day, students filter in at will; they don't have to cut today. Instead, they will review for the second exam as it suits them. Lisa stands before Mr. Bones (the articulated skeleton), holding hands with him.

"Scared Lovers Try Positions That They Can't Handle," she tells him while examining his wrist.

"What?" I ask.

"That's the eight wrist bones: scaphoid, lunate, triquetrum, pisiform, trapezium, trapezoid, capitate, hamate," she says. Med students have used such mnemonic devices for generations; many of them are considerably more raunchy. Today a man describes the same bones with "PTL Sucks Horse Cocks Twice Today."

"So what does PTL mean?" someone asks.

" 'Praise the Lord,' you know, that TV evangelism stuff."

"Yeah, or Pass the Loot," another responds. In today's news televangelist Jim Bakker is sentenced to forty-five years in prison and a $500,000 fine.

Mnemonics, repetition, touching and naming the parts—whatever it takes. The next exams are Monday, the morning written and the afternoon practical as before. The students know the drill and scramble to cover the learning objectives of six dissections. Those who got low grades are, of course, determined to do better. Over the next thirty minutes, they keep arriving, and soon the room is full and buzzing with clusters of six students around each of the six cadavers.

While still referring to the lecture they just heard, the students also make syntheses with books, Mr. Bones, X rays posted in the rooms and the hallway, the knowledge each student has (from the different dissections), and, of course, the cadaver on the table in their midst. I think of the Rembrandt painting, *The Anatomy Lesson of Dr. Tulp,* in which Dr. Tulp shows the muscles of the forearm. In this case, every student is a Dr. Tulp. Dr. Rizzolo walks into the room twice, available for questions, but the students take no notice of him: they are too busy learning from each other.

There is one other source of information: the bodies of the students. As they discuss the structures of the hands, for example, they hold up their own and poke at them, pull fingers forward and back. Pete shows Jonathan how to extend the thumb away from the hand so that the abductors that make up part of the "anatomical snuffbox" become clear. (See Figure 20 above.)

"Hey, *dude!*" Jonathan exudes, poking his forefinger into the triangular dimple at the base of his thumb. "I can feel it now, two strands, just like in the cadaver. I couldn't feel them before, but they must have been there!"

Bill pulls a tendon in the forearm of the cadaver, causing the little finger, skinned and white, to pull back.

"See? The extensor indicis allows you to point your forefinger, but it also works the little finger."

"Hey, that's great. If only we could pull the tendons during the exam," someone says.

"Yeah, and the carpi ulnaris was what that guy didn't have in the lecture today," another points out, referring to the first patient Dr. Wolf presented.

Some critics have said that the anatomy course is the first step in dehumanizing the body, leading physicians to see patients only as scientific exhibits. While depersonalization is certainly a problem in medicine—anyone who has waited a long time at an office or clinic will agree to that—I don't think, based on what I've seen here, that anatomy courses should take the blame. I can't comment on other labs, other programs, other instructors, but I hope they also allow students to make many connections between the implied personhood of the cadavers, the students's own bodies, and future patients. If anything, the cadavers here receive doses of empathy, not objectification. When Bill pulls the cadaver's tendon he is, in a sense, "reanimating" that body. Momentarily and hypothetically, the flesh of that hand regains action and suggests the delicacy and power of all human hands. The students' awareness of hands is growing, in part because they dissect them into parts, but also because they see the dynamic complexity of the whole hand.

"It's amazing how the hand works," Pete says to me at Table 1, shaking his head in wonder. "It is a long time in getting to it, with all the cutting and trimming, but after eight hours or so, you start to get some real payback on how it all works. And when you explain it to your buddies, you really start to feel confident that you understand it." As the students question each other, add details, and settle disagreements with the text, they build a corporate narrative; it is corporate in the sense of communal, but it is also corporate in a root sense of "having to do with the body." We might say that a corpus of knowledge arises from the corpses. Or we might say it is embodied or even incarnated knowledge. Each student has the motivation to remember some version of this story for at least three reasons: the impending exam, the future use of such information in medical practice, and the intrinsic interest to see "how it all works."

For about ninety minutes the room has a quiet buzz, punctuated by occasional laughter. I hear phrases drifting by:

". . . and remember these all anastomose to each other . . ."

". . . this medially rotates . . ."

". . . if you damage his nerve, these muscles are affected . . ."

One student carries a volume entitled *Clinical Anatomy Made Ridiculously Simple.*

". . . that's medial, not median . . ."

". . . let me perturb your balance . . ." (borrowing Dr. Wolf's terminology from his lectures).

One student draws the musculature of a finger on the board, chalk in one hand, scalpel in the other.

". . . remember, the kidneys are retroperitoneal . . ."

". . . it doesn't necessarily have to synapse there . . ."

". . . so the ulnar nerve does the same thing on both sides of the hand?"

I lean against the sinks and watch them talk. They are now miles ahead of me in anatomical knowledge, out of my league! It is entirely clear to me that I will never be a doctor, regardless of any fantasies I have entertained. I would need some pre-med science classes, admission to med school, and a residency—probably about ten years of my life. Do I even have that long? My dad didn't when he was my age. Furthermore, I'd probably make a lousy doctor; I'd better stick to teaching and writing.

I also know that this isn't my social cohort. Some of the students will invite me to their class Halloween party, but I feel that it should be their party by themselves. Furthermore, the irrepressible Jonathan keeps asking me to introduce him to my college-aged daughter, making very clear what generation I belong to. So where am I? I'm suspended between the students' generation of emerging professionals and my father's generation, some of whom, like him, are dead. While I hope that my own career will continue to evolve, I will keep on teaching and writing. But I also have to consider the end of my life as well and ask: what things do I want to do in the ever-shrinking time I have? My dad died at age fifty-six, a number I am now slowly approaching, and with some trepidation. If I follow his lead, I don't have much time left—not to mention the drunken driver who may, on any evening, careen across the highway's white line.

I have always felt that the ideal teachers are, in a sense, dispensable, because their major aim should be to make students independent learners. My dad's last lessons occurred after his death, when he was a totally passive teacher, letting students make their own discoveries amongst his tissues and bones, matching up such terms as I'm hearing in the background. This teaching may have been some of his finest work, his greatest gift.

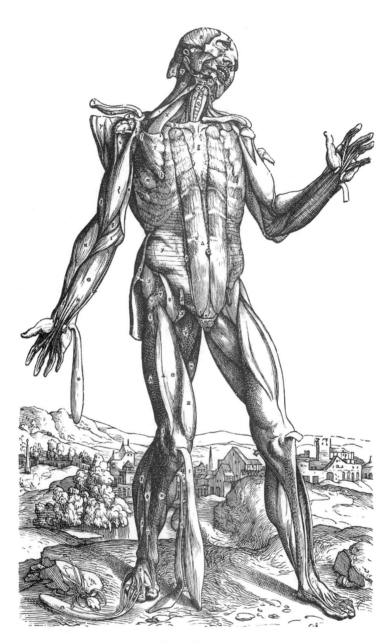

THE BICEPS

(Figure 21)

From *De fabrica*, The Fifth Plate of the Muscles, page 184.

THE BICEPS (the "two-headed" muscle) is labeled by the Greek letter zeta ("ζ") on the cadaver's right arm. The short head of the biceps ("b") attaches to the coracoid prominence of the scapula. The long head arches by means of a tendon ("f"—obscure) over the head of the humerus and attaches to another part of the scapula.

Dissection has removed the most prominent muscles of the torso. The twin rectus abdominis muscles (on either side of the navel) are extended too high for humans, all the way to the first rib (instead of the fifth, sixth, and seventh ribs, considerably lower); other mammals, as Vesalius knew, have this higher attachment.

THE GROSSER THE BETTER

• • •

THE SECOND REVIEW session, and the full class is present. Dr. English starts the review hour, as I sit in the back row with Steve, Jonathan, and Margaret. English reviews the place and times for the lab practical and puts up the four groups with the times.

Compared to the first review session five weeks before, this is a festive occasion. Ten of the fifteen dissections are done. Since all the students passed the first written and lab exams, they know what they are doing and what to expect in the lab, and Dr. English tells them so.

"You did a great job on the first exam," he says. "If you've been keeping up, this one should go well too. We'll have twenty-five questions, including two X rays. We're also dreaming up something interesting for a surface anatomy station." The phrase "surface anatomy" is literally a paradox, since anatomy, strictly speaking, has to do with cutting into the volume of bodies. Surface anatomy — external body landmarks such as "bony prominences" or grooves between muscles — doesn't take up much time in this class, although a $9.75 paperback on the topic is available in the bookstore. Nonetheless the concept is important, since patients always present their surface anatomy.

Dr. English describes a scheduling problem and asks the students to vote on two possible solutions. The students seem to appreciate the courtesy of his request and the shared decision-making: he treats them more like colleagues than students to be ordered around. The students are much more quiet during this review session; there are none of the called-out comments like last time, Freudian attacks, or nervous humor.

"Okay, let's zoom through some slides," English says, and the familiar paired slides flash onto two screens in the front. As before, one slide shows a labeled anatomical specimen, while the other screen shows a typewritten question and five choices. The slides look bright red, as if in life—*red meat*—and I ask a nearby instructor about their color. "Latex injection," he informs me.

The parade goes more slowly than English's verb *zoom* suggests, and we have plenty of time to analyze the slide and the possible answers. As before, we have about fifteen questions with a variety of structures (muscles, nerves, veins and arteries, bones, cartilage), and then a second trip through, with English's commentary on how to answer such questions. He also points out how these questions are similar to the questions on the national board exams these students will be taking at the end of their second year of med school.

While discussing an arm-movement question, English says, "Be sure to supinate your hand while removing a wine cork, so that your powerful biceps muscle comes into play." The students pay attention to English's comment, and some make the motion of drawing the hand up with the thumb outward. If you feel your biceps (the muscle in the front of your upper arm—perhaps the most famous muscle of the body, as in the traditional phrase "to make a muscle"), you can feel it contract during this motion. (See Figure 21 above.) The pleasant notion of opening a wine bottle helps give the right mood for remembering. Is opening a bottle of wine—a gift for guests perhaps—anything like opening a cadaver for wisdom?

The last slide shows the skeletal bones of the hand, wrist, and lower (or "distal") forearm. An arrow indicates the largest bone in the wrist, the capitate (which means "head," basically the head portion at the end of the two forearm bones). When the slide flashed up for the first time, I heard scattered but intense chuckles; seeing students fingering their wrists and moving their mouths, I imagine them using the PTL mnemonic.

"So you all got that one, right?" English asks them. "In my day it was

'Never Lower Tillie's Pants—Grandmother Might Come Home.' The bones weren't any different then, but the names were."

I mention the PTL version to Dr. Wolf.

"That's pretty tame, actually. All mine were considerably grosser, and that's why they worked. The grosser the better. I remember some of them today—fourteen years later," he says.

I think about mnemonics I have heard, such as "Ten Zebras Bit My Cock" (for the nerves of the face). Why is grosser better? There may be several factors. One, certainly, is a kind of personal creativity at work, a rebellion even, against the classical authority of all the other terms in the lecture and text. In a "gross" mnemonic, the student takes charge and brings her/his own energy and creativity to the structures. Furthermore, the use of short, Anglo-Saxon words—instead of the long scientific words of Greek or Latin origin—gives a domestication that makes the structures more local, less foreign. That some of the words are "dirty" gives further energy, memorability, and humor. The exaggerated grossness is whimsically inappropriate, a kind of play. But there is also, I feel, a release of anger and disgust about the oppressive features of the anatomy lab, the anatomical discipline, and perhaps even the total rigors of medical school. Maybe some students dislike their increasing intimacy with the cadavers? The gross mnemonic device becomes an act of vengeance, a "cutting down to size" of anatomical terms, goals, structures. (Charles LeBaron's book comes to mind: *Gentle Vengeance: An Account of the First Year of Harvard Medical School.* LeBaron says very little about his anatomy course, however.)

There may be one more factor, at least in some of the mnemonics, a kind of reanimation going on, an eroticization of dead material. "Sacred Lovers Try Positions That They Can't Handle" brings life to dead bones, a comic energy coupling the lovers of the mnemonic and, in another sense, the students and the wrist bones. I think of a touching nature film showing a troop of elephants crossing a grassy field. When an old, female elephant suddenly collapsed and died, her comrades crowded around her, trying to nudge her back to life. The last, desperate act was the attempt of the oldest male to mount her sexually. None of these attempts worked, and when her herd gradually realized her life was gone, they began to move without her. Those elephants (and these students) seek to project vitality onto dead flesh, and, in so doing, they affirm their own living existence. "Let's get this straight," the mnemonics and other forms of humor seem to say, "you, the cadavers, are dead—although we can imagine your past life—but we who work on you today are very much alive."

My dad would have loved even the vilest of mnemonics. He had a great sense of humor and, like many of his generation, struggled heroically to cast off the Victorian strictures of his parents. I sincerely hope that the student anatomists said a lot of strange and funny things over his body and that, on some eerie karmic level, he heard them.

CORPSES DON'T GET SORE

. . .

S ECOND LABORATORY EXAM. No one is dressed up—the students wear jeans and running or tennis shoes. I see half a dozen baseball caps. Are these symbols of independence, of confidence, or of a message, such as *We'd rather be somewhere else?*

As before, the students gather in batches by the fourth-floor elevator. This time, however, they are not silent, waiting and wondering in awe. They chatter away with outbursts of raucous laughter. I can easily hear them from some 100 feet away, around the corner and down the hall; I recognize laughs of particular students. As groups of students come by for the exam, many exchange greetings with me. Although Cliff says, on his way by, "Like cows to the slaughter," none of them look in the least cowed.

It's the "cafeteria-style" exam again, with twenty-five exhibits and three or four rest stations, depending on the size of each group. One rest station is in the hall near the embalming tank where a lab coordinator runs the timer and where I make my notes. I amuse myself by seeing how many students wear wedding rings, assuming that some may take them off for dissection.

Before or after the exam (and even during it), several students ask me whether I have seen the current film *Gross Anatomy*. I haven't; have they? About half of them have seen it. They generally feel that it is a formulaic B movie, but they are glad that someone has paid attention to their work, even on that level. (Evidently there is a certain loneliness to "busting your ass" as a med student—*Who really cares?* they sometimes feel.) One student actually likes the movie a lot: "It's a good facsimile, but you have to be a med student to really enjoy it." For him, the movie is a validation, and a statement of things he has perhaps felt but not articulated. I think he also senses that the world of anatomy lab, where people cut into cadavers, is closed and privileged—his realm of knowledge and power. At the same time, I think he wants people to know what he is experiencing.

A student has clipped out the newspaper advertisement for the film and taped it to Art English's door, with a few changes. *Gross Anatomy* is changed to *Human Anatomy* (reflecting this course's title) and the line "No one thought a rebel like Joe Slovak would make it through med school" had "Joe Slovak" crossed out and *Art English* written in. It seems, indirectly, a tribute to Art and the course. I'm not sure when it went up, but since Dr. English hasn't taken it down, it appears that he accepts the compliment.

The students move from station to station in intervals of one minute and fifteen seconds. One woman nonchalantly blows gum into big yellow bubbles. As before, all students wear their lab coats, but no gloves.

While they take the exam, I look over a copy of the questions. Of twenty-five questions, about half are straight identification, such as "identify the tagged structure." These are the "see-and-say" questions of the ethos: *Let's get oriented; let's isolate this structure; let's apply the name.* The other half are more relational or functional: "The tagged structure receives its blood supply from/is innervated by . . ." Thus both naming and seeing relationships continue to be important to the examiners. Some of the students who made their presentations dynamic or dramatic may have an advantage over their colleagues who only identified the structures.

I ask Larry Rizzolo, who is monitoring the exam, whether a superficial anatomy question was set up.

"Yes, well, it's a hand, with a nerve-supply question."

"Not a real person?"

"No. We used to do that, but the person would get sore over the three or four hours."

So: dead people do a better job at this kind of work. As I walk through the exhibits later, when the exam is over, I see all the muscles, veins, and joints displayed—tagged and well lit—remaining like this for the entire time since the exam was set up and, of course, during the exam itself, at least thirty hours.

Here is a cadaver on his back, his knee bent up. The kneecap is pulled back, revealing the inner joint with the polished meniscuses that cover the tops of the lower leg bones. A short structure ties the joint together right across the middle, on a slant. It's the posterior cruciate ligament, one of two that cross in the middle of the knee. The question asks what kind of movement this structure limits, so that the knee doesn't bend too far. Certainly a live person couldn't provide this exhibit.

The surface anatomy question, it turns out, refers to a single hand, severed at the wrist and swaddled in cloth. Although clearly gray and dead, this hand still has enough humanness about it to be disturbing as it sits on the white enamel tray. If there is an "end of the road," this hand has surely reached it.

INTIMACIES OF THE ANATOMY LAB

• • •

(SECOND ESSAY)

NAKED BODIES, UNDEFENDED postures, bare genitals. All these make us think of sexual intimacy, especially in a culture that often reduces physical intimacy to sexual activity. Since "to sleep with someone" has come to mean to have sexual intercourse, we fail to have words for the gently intimate act of actually sleeping with someone, and we tend to lose awareness of other senses of intimacy. The anatomy lab is not, with its sights and smells, a sexy place. Old dead people would be a turn-on only for necrophiliacs, I suppose, a thought that gives me the creeps. There is intimacy with the cadavers, yes, but it is not sexual. There is also growing intimacy within the class of students at work here and in the other classes where they see each other. The students are becoming closer as a social cohort. At first they were emotionally paralyzed by the strangeness of this place; as they gained confidence and created their own social stability, they more and more discussed all the topics of their generation: music, food, films, cars, trouble with landlords, who's attractive, who's dating whom, and the like. When only men are talking, there's now very specific discussion of the attractions of female classmates. One female cutter explained that she did an internship with a researcher who was not only good scientifically but personally "hot." In other words, sexual topics do, in fact, enter the lab, but only as they are brought here by the vital world of the students. No one—at least in my hearing—has talked about the sexual nature of the cadavers.

And yet there are various intimacies in the lab and even a sense of *eros* in the lab that deserve discussion.

The word *intimacy* has, in its Latin root, the meanings of "inner," "inwardness," and "innermost." The related word *intima* in anatomy refers to the innermost layer (or coat or "tunica") of both artery and vein; each of us has hundreds of miles of intima in our bodies. Such inner structures suggest a sense of innerness, the most remote of tissues—as if you could get to the heart or the bottom of a person by dissection, to the very innermost part of his or her being. This urge is important in the motivation of med students, who want to learn how human beings, *at base,* are put together. We might call this a mechanical intimacy.

Such mechanical intimacy, however, is not highly valued in this culture, which pretty much ignores the inner workings of the body. Most of us don't know about the intimal layer of our blood vessels—or much else under the skin. Our modern society is so estranged from the human bodies in which we dwell that our corporeality becomes a kind of paradox, a locus of conflicting attitudes. While the body is an icon, a sign of health, of sex, of athleticism, something we are fascinated with to the point of idolatry, it is also in some ways a taboo subject, a collection of cells that carries us around and ultimately betrays us, in sickness and eventual death. Much of our advertising centers on images of healthy young men and women, but we have little idea of how their health works, why their body parts and shapes are alluring, or even the cultural determinants of our attitudes (why we currently favor low subdermal fat, long torsos, wide shoulders, etc.). Our sense of living in the body is minimal, despite years of "physical education," which typically teaches rules of games and particular skills, but rarely any in-depth understanding of the body systems and how to care for them. Ask people to point to their spleen, and they'll have no idea where it is. Ask them what the liver does—the largest gland in the body—and they will most likely not know.

Who stole our bodies? There are many and pervasive sources of our alienation from our bodies: Greek idealism (the noble Platonic forms versus the imperfect embodiments), Cartesian dualism (the wonderful mind versus the gross matter of the body), religious dualism (exalted spirit versus the sinning body), academic rationalism (the intelligent mind versus the stupid body), and even capitalism (personal career and wealth versus the impediments of the body). The body has become the dross, the dregs, the work of the devil. Small wonder we have trouble knowing and enjoying the bodies we live in! And small tragedy, too, since our ignorance of diet and the effects of stress makes us less healthy.

Meanwhile, modern society avoids dealing directly with death, with dead persons, with the realities of failing bodies, or with a public health system that might improve the health of millions of people, rich and poor. While all students probably have experienced death in their families, many or most have not seen someone die or a body being prepared for burial—routine occurrences in previous times. Some may never have attended a funeral. Thus the denial of corporality in our culture touches both the living body and the dead.

If cutting is a way into the body, what do we find when we get there, and what is our relationship to this dark inner volume? What is this voyage within, with all its sensuous glory? The journey is dramatic: cuts are kinetic actions, commitments of mind and body to make the scalpel or probe work within the tissues as active bodies meet inert ones. The senses perceive this concrete intimacy: the students *feel* the shapes and textures of skin and bone, muscles and tendons, nerve and blood vessels; they *see* the colors and densities of the tissues; they *smell* the formaldehyde; they *hear* the tearing of adhesions and the sawing or cracking of the bones. To work your way into the body is to come to know its textures and qualities through direct, sensory apprehension in a way that our touch-aversive society otherwise avoids or even forbids. The cut is a specialized kind of touch, one that destroys in order to promote understanding.

Another paradox is this: the deeper you cut, the more you *do not* find some inner magical secret. There is, as Richard Selzer found, no "exact location of the soul" to be found through technical cutting. He concludes that such a soul will be found by one kind of vision: "only the poet, for he sees what no one else can. He was born with the eye for it" (*Mortal Lessons*, p. 70).

If there is understanding to be gained, it may run like this: with no single inner center of life to discover, life is to be perceived everywhere in the body, in every bone, fiber, and tendril, and furthermore, as a process, not an object, even in the mundane act of walking—which uses some 200 muscles, a zillion nerves and blood vessels, our bones, our skin, our nutritional resources, our hormones, our brain, our intentions, our ideas, our emotions, and more. The good physician, therefore, deals with the whole patient, not just one sick organ or system. The students have touched the heart and the pelvis already, without finding the essence of life. Perhaps the head still tempts them? The uncovering of the brain itself is not far off. In the traditional phrase, the whole of human is more than the sum of the parts. I recall a sentence of Buckminster Fuller's: "I seem to be a verb." Maybe the phrase "human bodies" can be other than adjective and noun; how about noun and verb, as in "human bodies or embodies," meaning that to be human is to live in a body? Back to the soul: can a human body *body* without the physical casing? Or does a soul *soul,* without need of a body? If I had a direct line to my father at this point, I know he would tell me.

Another sense of intimacy is in the tracing and clarification. As the students pick fat, separate structures, and trace them through various tissues, they see the innerness of the connective vasculature, nerves, and tendons; they see the works, the webs, the machinery, the electrical systems, the "backstage" of the human body. Over and over, I see the students appreciating the body, *appreciating* in its original sense of "knowing the worth," an immense wealth of value here. From the chaotic scraps, names, and tangles slowly emerges the genius of structure, or abstract design, or organic interrelationship, for which the students express their wonder and awe. When students at Table 1 show Jonathan the "anatomical snuffbox" at the base of the thumb, he delights in perceiving the deployment of the tendons that work the thumb. *So that's how it works!* is a thrill of recognition.

There is also the giving of names (like Fred, Rose, and Job) to the cadavers that expresses and creates a more general relationship between cutter and cadaver. We've seen the student jargon as well as the strictly anatomical nomenclature. All three of these namings participate in an ancient tradition known as word magic: in folk tales (for example "Rumpelstiltskin"), in scripture (the naming of the animals in Genesis), and, generally, in the "discovery" and naming of lands and even in the baptism of children; to give a name to (or to learn the name of) an artery, a nerve, a lymphatic duct is to have a sense of familiarity, perhaps even ownership or control. When Lisa says, "This is right atrium," she knows the structure, puts the phrase to it, and sows this seed of knowledge into the minds of her listeners. "I'm finding all sorts of things . . . but which ones are they?" says Steve. His job is not over until object and word have been put together.

Can familiarity, either by word usage or the hours of cutting, breed contempt? Yes—at least at times. Students tire of their cadavers, the work, the rigorous approach; they express their disgust, sadness, and tedium directly, or through humor. But they keep coming back to the lab, because there are rewards of discovery beyond such contempt.

Is there a danger in that, through this naming process, each structure becomes converted into or reduced to anatomical language, "scientized" or "medicalized" (in Ivan Illich's terms)? Perhaps so, and perhaps such a disciplined perception is a necessary risk for medical work. The trick for each physician, therefore, will be to develop technical understanding without losing the human wisdom that will also be a part of his or her ability to heal. Some of these other layers of meaning and value are evident in alternate names the students develop, that will never appear in the *Nomina anatomica*. The student mnemonics and slang ("puppy," "PTL," "birdbath," "the bowel from hell") build bridges between object and self, the formal and the familiar, the unknown and the known.

I hear students using language to explore the past humanity of their cadavers: how did they die, what were their final months or years like, what distinctive body build or evidence of illness do the cadavers display? In these observations and words are kernels of stories, thumbnail biographies— speculative, of course, but indicative of a kind of intimacy between student and specimen. These stories have grown in the last few weeks, a contrast to the early part of the course, when the humanity of the cadaver was studiously avoided; then, the strategy was to cover the body almost completely, to render it a biological exhibit only. But when Karl and Stephen look at the cut on the cadaver's jaw, they can sketch a possible narrative for this man's death. When Gail and Lisa make up a presentation with their cadaver in running shoes, they are using narrative activity as a way of showing the kind of life process the cadaver once performed.

Conversely, there was another kind of intimacy of language that modern anatomists have pretty much demolished, the use of eponyms, or the naming of a structure after the discoverer. The "Eustachian tube" is now generally known as the "auditory tube." ("The Circle of Willis," a system of connecting arteries at the base of the brain, is one of the few surviving phrases.) While some medical history and tributes to the discoverers are lost through this purging, the descriptive names are clearer and easier to learn.

With the difficult work of the pelvis past, the students have now dissected all the large volumes of the torso. By dealing with the sexual organs, and by listening to the lecture on childbirth, another difficult area has been confronted and, on many levels, understood. In "popping" the pelvis, the students have survived one of the harshest anatomical moves, and have become, at least on a symbolic level, part of the childbirth ritual, a maieutics of anatomical wisdom. In a mythic sense, the anatomy course takes us from death to birth, and back to death. To experience and assess these transits is to gain a lot of experience fast.

The social linking of the students, especially the teams that cut together, is yet another kind of intimacy. Each working group takes on its own dynamics, emergent leaders, and clowns. While the students know each other from other classes and other contexts I don't share, I enjoy watching their growing familiarity as they work together, teach each other, make jokes, endure the tedium, and more. With five twenty-hour dissections together, each set of lab partners builds a community of cooperating learners; they help each other become doctors. As they overlap with other sets, comparing working methods and discoveries, they become veterans of shared experience, comrades in arms who have survived the same trials, who have taken steps toward a common goal.

Furthermore, there are seeds of future professional behavior: when one student helps another with a dissecting problem, she or he is doing a preliminary version of a "consult," a medical referral that is important professionally (and economically) in medical practice.

As the students work, they sometimes lean on each other or put an arm on a neighboring shoulder. They are becoming a cohort, a group of persons going through a long, hard process together. They share the same stresses, self-doubts, fatigue, feelings of inadequacy before overloads of assignments, but they make their way forward and they draw strength from each other. They are no longer pre-meds, competing with each other (and anyone else), but colleagues who will all become physicians, if they endure. They are forming the new class of a guild, a group of professionals who have trained hard and long, have gone through rites of passage and certification, and who at last have, in the traditional phrase, rights and responsibilities. (I have heard some carping and rivalry as well, which will also be part of their professional world.)

The instructors are part of this process, although at a certain remove. They are teachers, of course, but also cheerleaders, encouragers, and supporters. They treat the students as future physicians, using phrases like, "You are likely to see this in your practice." Dr. Wolf's joke about the medical pecking order is a kind of avuncular intimacy, a shared recognition of social levels within the profession.

As I get to know the students better, they talk with me more and more. One reason is that I am a neutral figure, detached from the institution. But while conversational intimacy grows between me and many of the students, I know that we are separating professionally: they are racing by me in their detailed understanding of the body. I am somewhat jealous of their growth and their future niche within the adepts of medicine, but I realize my role is different, and I wish them success on their way and, in a sense, wave goodbye. I cannot join their society professionally or socially.

When Lisa looks forward to "all of this" being over and committed to memory, she's referring largely to the mental control of the information. Spending more than a hundred hours with a dead body is an undeniable invitation to understand mortality and the ultimate terminus for every human being. While the anatomy course doesn't do much with these questions, student conversation makes some explorations, and, later, the Service of Reflection and Gratitude will offer its contribution. As the students visit more tables, they see and consider many of the ways human lives can come to an end. In a personal way, the students are maturing at an accelerated rate, almost like "forced" flowers. They are becoming veterans or, at least on one level, "experts" (the word means, at root, "experienced") during this intense sixteen weeks in the lab. It's a lot to ask of anyone, particularly with all their other courses, but the students not only do it, they seem to thrive on it. "That's so cool!" I hear them exclaim as they look into their cadavers. What is a living human being? A collection of many parts and systems that interrelate in such an elegant and powerful way that life is clearly more than the sum of the parts. Perhaps this insight has its fullest power to a person who has dissected a human body.

Beneath the cuts, the tracing, the names, the touching, the shared experience, and the expansion of consciousness, there is an underlying power, perhaps the deepest source of intimacy, a *fascination for flesh* that can be immediately satisfied by touch, inspection, and understanding. The power is evident in every action of the students as they cut and in the inspiration that comes to them through discoveries within the cadavers. In this developing bond I see a kind of eros, a love of the human body. Something primal happens in the lab, as primal as the Aztec priest removing the heart. There is a kind of animal passion *to know someone thoroughly,* an urge we most readily identify with sexual activity (especially with the biblical sense of knowing carnally) but an urge that may be worked out consciously and deliberately here, through a kind of protracted minuet (and not a danse macabre), much like the forceps and scissors of Dr. Margeson, as he metallically danced his way through the psoas muscle. The severity of the discipline of anatomy—the terms, the memorization, the grasping of spatial and functional relationships—provides a classical structure for the almost anarchic activity of tearing a body apart (the *sparagmos,* or tearing asunder of the body as in Euripides' play *The Bacchae*). The sixteen weeks are, in a sense, an extended lovemaking to one human body—an anatomical necrophilia in the most positive sense—and, by symbolic extension, to all human bodies. Even sexual experience seems a narrow (however powerful) band of experience in comparison with the carnal intimacy of anatomical dissection.

Eating the dead—perhaps the ultimate intimacy—has figured in many societies, even in the Christian communion. The students have kept alive a theme of necrophagia, partly as a joke, partly as a reflection of the actual bits of the cadaver flying into an unlucky mouth, partly as a profound symbolic tribute: the cadavers enter their memories as surely as a good meal enters their stomachs and becomes part of their bodies.

I think this sense of eros is one of the reasons students find the anatomy course one of the clearest rites of passage. The students, at the end of the course, are more ready for the intimacies of the consulting room. They are aware that a dead person has given them a body to take apart, a profound gift. As they grow in their estimation of this gift, they carry a sense of reverence and responsibility to future encounters with bodies, those of their living patients. When I go to my physician—or to a doctor I don't know at all, a specialist to whom I have been referred—the basic questions I carry are the following: Is there something seriously wrong with me? Will this doctor listen to me and treat me like a human being? Can he or she help me? My hope is that the sensitivity and wonder that can arise from dissection of a human body will not be beaten out of doctors by future training, professional stress, institutional imperatives, or years of routine. Here's what I'd like to say: "Hello, Dr. Z. You don't know me, but my body is just as wonderful as the cadaver you dissected your first year of med school. Of course, I am alive now, and, because of that, I feel worry and fear about my health. Please comfort and help me."

As I walk to work, I pass through woods animated by squirrels. They pick nuts from the ground and race up tree trunks to eat them. Sometimes bits of husk fall on my path or onto my face as I walk below; I catch some of this tiny shrapnel in my hand and see the precise marks of squirrel teeth. They are anatomists of their own sort, accurately cutting to reach the parts that nourish them. At other times, they make arcing leaps across the ground, stop, look around, and *digdigdig* with the forepaws; they drop the nut from their mouths into the hole, push and pat the earth, and dash away. I remember from grade school that squirrels forget some of their buried treasures, which sometimes sprout and grow from this inadvertent planting. Similarly the students find nuts of knowledge and deposit these in their brains for future use. Some insights and facts will be easily recovered. Some will be forgotten. The neglected seeds will not sprout a tree, but there are other by-products of dissection: the students gain ability in learning, intuitions about the genius of the body, and personal confidence that they can deal with complex information, the mechanical intricacies of the human body, and even with death itself.

PART III

FROM CADAVER TO CARCASS TO REINCORPORATION

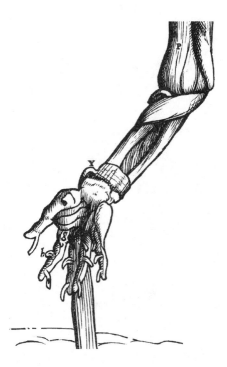

The Lumbricals

(Figure 22)

From *De fabrica,* The Seventh Plate of the Muscles, detail, page 190.

ON THIS HIGHLY dissected right hand, the lumbricals stick out ("g," and possibly "h"). These tiny muscles derive their name from a Latin word meaning "worm," because of their shape. Saunders and O'Malley warn, however, "that too much attention should not be paid to the small muscles of the hand [in this woodcut] since they were grouped in a manner quite foreign to modern conceptions" (page 104).

YOU GUYS HAVE YOUR GUTS?

• • •

WHAT'S THIS? STUDENTS are standing on the sidewalk outside the anatomy building, *just visiting.* I haven't seen this all semester, but today is the day after the exams, and students are, for once, taking it easy. Some actually sit on the grass, lolling and lazing. I join them to chat and watch still others slowly straggle in to campus, having slept through one or more classes.

"Last time, I just went home and went to sleep. This time, we had all kinds of parties," various ones report. The freshman medical class is more of a social entity now, and the period of abstinence for study and examination needs appropriate restitution! I see Jonathan picking up his mail, and we catch up briefly. He is scheduled to be in the lab this afternoon, so I dutifully ask him whether I'll see him up there.

"Naaaa," he replies with a grin. "I'm going to be miles away."

Others are distant as well: attendance at the lecture is light, barely half the class. Lois Wolf does a good job with "Manual Muscle Testing," especially the opening slides. She has paste-ups of various bodies (flabby, muscleman, female) with the superposition of the head of her husband (Steve Wolf, one of the anatomy professors) smiling absurdly. The students laugh uproariously, aware that Steve knows that some silliness has been afoot, but not its exact contents. He himself is hundreds of miles away, in Phoenix, Arizona, for a convention—helpless against such satire. Lois Wolf tells us about manual muscle testing. While various high-tech machines can give readings of muscle strength (torque, velocity, average torque, maximal torque), even with computerized printouts, a physical therapist (she is one) or a physician can use hands only to get an idea of the strength of a muscle or muscle group. Such knowledge can aid diagnosis (particularly the location of nerve injury), therapy, and referral. She shows us a videotape of various patients and their compromised musculature: some are in wheelchairs, and one has trouble walking because of a dragging foot. In many cases, these conditions can be alleviated by applications of anatomical knowledge. She doesn't mention it, but wise physicians often touch their patients—on the arm, say, as greeting, as a sign of intimacy, as a symbol of solace. I've gone on rounds in the hospital with my family physician; he makes it a point to touch each patient in friendship. I remember a study from many years ago in which researchers asked workers in a library to touch fingers with some patrons as they checked out books but to avoid the fingers of the others. This difference was coded, and interviewers asked all patrons about their experience in the library, how their work went, whether they were happy, and so on. Those whose fingers had been touched routinely reported more positive feelings about their visit. Isn't this a truth we all know? Why, then, do we so carefully avoid touching each other?

I think about these matters as I take the stairs upstairs. The labs are not crowded today. A dozen students are in the hall, craning their necks toward the key for the lab exam posted on the bulletin board. There is the usual chorus of groans and cheers. In each dissecting room, only a handful of students are cutting, David and Cliff among them. They are finishing up the hand dissection, while Larry and John at Table 1 and Keith and Bill, at Table 5, go ahead to the leg and foot. The students continue the discussion of the exams for a while.

"They never even mentioned the word *infra*," complains one.

"Did you hear about old Todd?" another asks. "He couldn't get oriented on one exhibit, so he looked around for any lab instructors, then put his right hand on the head to see if there was a nose or not." All the heads were covered so that folds of cloth masked facial features; Todd's hand, ungloved at the time, would have been making a bold gesture of familiarity and inquiry—not to mention breaking the exam rules.

One woman mentions the preserved hand exhibit. "It had fingernail polish on! Did you see?" Others joke about the roving hand in the movie *Addams Family Values.*

Conversation moves quickly on to a variety of topics from sports to movies but turns to Halloween, and specifically to a med student party tonight. The students talk about their costumes and joke about the anatomy lab's appropriateness for Halloween. Some have invited me to come to the party, but I feel that such camaraderie is rightly theirs, not mine.

Today is indeed October 31, the Evening of All Hallows Day, when saints are remembered. I have thought of my father as a saint, not during my oedipal conflict years, of course, but as I later watched him endure his medical trials I thought of him as earning his sainthood. He decided early on to thank anyone for any favor, to avoid complaining, and to bear his trials with patience and, when possible, good cheer. The following—and related—day, is November 2, or All Souls Day, when all the dead are honored and properly put to rest. To the more popular mind, the ghosts dance a "danse macabre" before daybreak catches them and sends them back to their graves. It's a harvest festival, not only for the souls, who, one way or another, are gathered up, but also for the summer crops. For many communities, it was the end of summer produce and the beginning of winter hunting, the chasing of live game. So we still have the ritual symbols of corn candy, pumpkins, and bobbing for apples. For the moderns, Daylight Savings Time ends, and the evenings are suddenly much darker, a quick jump toward winter's shorter days, often a time of study and the practice of crafts to pass the long, dreary months. The dead in this anatomy lab are part of the summer's harvest, which will be ritually celebrated by the Service of Reflection and Gratitude. The students now hunt for wisdom of muscle and sinew in this carefully given, carefully preserved flesh.

"We gotta wet her down," Cliff says, looking at Little Old Lady. She has been drying over the past several days, especially in her thin arms. On one wrist, skinned down to sinew and bone, her plastic wristband still slides up and down; on it is the number identifying her. Cliff carefully shakes the preserver bottle over her.

"You guys have your guts?" Larry Rizzolo asks, holding up a plastic bag.

"Yeah, right here," David says, holding up his bag.

"Okay, then these must go with this one," Rizzolo says, restoring the bowels to another table. I especially enjoy the phrase "your guts," not so much for the sense of the warm guts we all carry at the moment, pulsing lunch downward with their peristaltic waves, but for the sense of *belonging* that the cadaveric guts somehow assume during the dissection, belonging to the dissectors rather than to the bodies from which they are taken. "Your guts" are the guts that have been received as gifts, through touch, through concept, through insight—by each student.

"Look in here," Cliff urges me, and he shows me the inner arterial supply to the hand. Examples of "wisdom of the body" (Cannon's phrase), the high-pressure arteries are hidden deep, along or between bones, where they can't be readily slashed. The low-pressure veins, by contrast, often run on the surface of the body.

David is discussing the deep palmar arch with Dr. Margeson, who says that it "can be picked up on the ulnar side." David pokes around and locates the way into that space and shows it to me, but he says, "That's two seconds' worth to present, but it could take more than an hour to prepare." He is not going to dissect it.

Similarly, at Table 1, Larry and John have made some practical decisions. They are stripping the skin off the foot with unusual speed.

"What's the approach, guys?" I ask them.

"We realized that the slower way earned us sixes on the presentations all right, but the other guys were also getting sixes with a lot less work. We're taking more shortcuts now."

Rippp! Across the room there is a short but intense tearing sound.

"Ooops. What would that have been?" Bill says. He and his partner survey the facedown cadaver, with its foot grotesquely lying directly on its buttock; clearly something has given way in the knee to allow this. They look into this joint, already dissected, and find the torn ligament—the anterior cruciate—which has given way in the absence of other supports (such as the patellar tendon) that have already been cut.

"Yep, that makes sense. This would be the tendon that helps keep the knee from bending too much," Keith says.

"Right. We had the posterior cruciate on the lab exam," Bill says. (The question on the exam isolated the function of that tendon to keep the knee from hyperextending.)

"Well, we can sure skin the foot easier now."

"Just as I planned it!" Bill claims.

Back at Table 3, David is working deep on the hand. He shows me some of the muscles and tendons that work the fingers.

I ask him whether Little Old Lady was right- or left-handed.

"We think right-handed. The muscles are bigger here. These are the lumbricals," he says, showing me small muscles deep in the fingers of her right hand. "I think of them as the 'salute' muscles." A navy veteran, he makes a salute over his eyebrow, his fingers bowing up from the hand. "They are also important in writing, to push the pen away from the hand. I think she did a lot of writing. For the lumbricals, these are good-sized." (See Figure 22 above.)

Actual handwriting! Not typewriting, not word processing. What did she write? For whom? I think of my father, a man of letters who wrote much. Could the students who dissected him tell his trade?

As Cliff and David cut away, they hold hands with her, one hand holding, one hand cutting, trimming, probing. It seems to me that their young hands, vital and strong, receive an anatomic blessing from her dead hands, ancient and unraveling, stiff, but full of marvels.

I WANT TO CRY

• • •

CHAPLAIN DON SHOCKLEY has invited for lunch those med students who signed up to work on the Service of Reflection and Gratitude. We meet in a handsome room in the student center around a large square table formally set with tablecloths and flowers. Thirteen students are here, including two who rush over from the anatomy lab, where they have been readying their presentation on the hand for this afternoon.

He reads an excerpt from Lewis Thomas's *Lives of a Cell,* a passage about "bioacoustics," the multitude of noises in nature, most of which we never hear. The provocative words of this physician/essayist help to set the tone of appreciation for the complexities and richness of nature. While we eat lunch, Don tells us that the service has occurred yearly for the past nine years; it is different every year and primarily planned by the students. The service originated with a medical student who felt that something should be done at the end of the course for two reasons: (1) to finish the work not only anatomically but psychologically, and (2) to recognize the gift of the cadavers. Shockley mentions this history and says that usually about 80 to 90 percent of all first-year students come; evidently it has been important to them. Most of the faculty attend as well.

The purposes of the service, therefore, are twofold. First, the service should serve as a "ritual of disengagement," by which the students can reach some closure to the anatomical experience. "It doesn't seem appropriate to quit one day and just walk away from the table," he puts it. The service is primarily for the students, since the families of the cadavers have already had funeral or memorial services. Furthermore, the families may participate in yet another service at the end of the year when remains, in cremated form, are buried together (or returned to the family for their own burial service), he explains. The families are told that the students have such a service. Don says the families are pleased to know about the event.

The second purpose is to express gratitude for the chance to work closely with a donated body, to give thanks for the gift of this body to the donor. He says, "I have heard students ask, 'Did this person know he or she was going to end up here?' The answer is yes. They specifically left their bodies for the purpose of anatomical study or medical research.

"So that's the background and why we do the service. How does that sound?" Don asks the students.

"Very appropriate," says one, while the others nod assent and murmur their agreement.

"I want to cry," one woman sobs—I think. It's hard to make out her exact words, since she is already crying. Her neighbors pat her on the back and hand tissues to her.

Don acknowledges the emotions of the moment and says that as we work on the service some of that will disappear. In his words, "We'll get some emotional distancing on the service as we do the work of arranging it." Having sung at weddings and funerals of persons I know, I understand what he is saying. Part of the education of a physician is to know how and when to acknowledge emotions, how and when to give rein to them, how and when to be emotionally distanced. I have heard many people complain about physicians—often specialists—who seem uncaring and unfeeling, robots of sorts who can talk only in technical language. How has medical education failed them?

In the past, there has been music of different kinds. Don asks what musicians are in the class. Quickly the students identify a dozen or more possibilities. They evidently know each other well by now, and this particular group has many extroverted souls.

As they talk about the service, they also talk about their own feelings and questions, many stored up until today. As one man puts it, "I think a lot of us don't *really* think about what we are actually doing up there. We just kind of block it out."

"Do they specify uses of their bodies?" someone asks, and a series of questions about the donation of the bodies continues. Don answers all of these knowledgeably. (Much of the information is on a blue sheet provided at the beginning of the class; the students have either forgotten the information or weren't ready, at the time, to receive it.) There are two uses of the donated cadavers, teaching (as we have seen in the lab) and research. Some of the families hope that the gift will allow researchers to find a cure for the disease that caused the person's death, but the coordinators of the body program must patiently explain that such a discovery, from one cadaver, is not likely. For such families, the wish is a kind of a magical sentiment, a hopeful fantasy. The big breakthroughs in drugs, for example, come "up" through clinical trials on live animals, then on actual human patients; cadavers are not of any use in that work.

Since all the cadavers are provided through planned agreements, there are no unclaimed bodies, no bodies of derelicts, nor bodies that have been purchased, Don explains. (There are strange rumors that bodies are bought by med schools, as blood or plasma formerly were, but all three practices have officially ended.) All bodies in this lab have been given through a written agreement by the persons who have made this conscious choice. In America (and elsewhere), there have been abuses in the past—stolen bodies, exhumed bodies—but current supervision, legal provisions, and professional care of cadavers make such abuse just about impossible.

The rest of today's planning is to choose committees for music, text, and speakers. The students are quick to volunteer for responsibilities. One committee will deal with written statements from students. It will work like this: students may contribute written reflections, memories, narratives, journal entries, or poems. Some of these will be read during the service, and all of them will appear in a booklet provided to everyone at the service.

The 1:00 P.M. lecture is drawing near. The group plans to meet again in two weeks. I watch the students file out, ready to trade their meeting behavior for laboratory behavior. They will have many similar shifts in mood and function to make in their careers. I remember visiting an emergency room years ago in rural Washington state. I was far away from home and had a skin infection that was minor but painful and generally annoying. While I waited to be seen, a middle-aged man on an ambulance gurney was rushed past me; one of his work boots fell off by my chair. Eventually I was called back to the treatment area and cared for by a physician who, it turned out, had just worked on the ambulance patient, who had died from his heart attack. The physician, nonetheless, treated my minor problem with full attention and kindness. As I left, I saw the shape of a dead man beneath a sheet. In the waiting room his dusty boot still lay on its side.

NA NANA NA NA

• • •

THERE'S A GOOD crowd for the lecture today, perhaps representing some new resolves following the anatomy exam. I see a few male students who have rarely come to any of the recent lectures. Says one, "I missed too many questions on the lab practical! I guess there's the possibility some of them were discussed in lecture!"

The topic today, and for the next two lectures, is the neck—that narrow, unassuming stalk linking head and torso. But think of all the important structures running through there, carrying blood for the brain, nerves from the brain, food for the stomach, air for the lungs, as well as the muscles that turn and help support the head, and the vertebral column that holds the head upright. This is the crucial site for hanging or decapitation, whether by ax or guillotine. A beheading is an awesome and largely historical event, though we have a trace of it in an actor's bow as a symbolic offering of his or her head to the audience—previously a queen and king. The bow says, symbolically: *I am so in your debt, I offer the head that I know you could have chopped off at any moment; I serve at your pleasure.*

Larry Rizzolo is our speaker today. He has a sly sense of humor and a deadpan delivery. One day he got tangled in the microphone wire as he walked around the stage. Untangling the wire from his lab coat and long legs, he quipped, "Maybe I can follow this back to my mother."

Today he enlivens his discussion of anatomical triangles of the neck and their structures with slides of two shrews, tiny, mouselike creatures.

"How many cervical [neck] vertebrae?" he asks.

"Seven," the students immediately reply; evidently they have heard this one before.

Next a slide of a giraffe flashes up.

"How many?"

"Seven!" they yell.

"Right."

Rizzolo continues with his formal slides of the human neck, and a few die-hards call out "Seven," once more. Whatever the physical length, the necks of mammals generally have seven bones. The shrews and giraffes are this instructor's "wake-up slides."

Near the end of the talk, a slide shows two actors, one portraying Count Dracula, the other Ripe Young Maiden, with neck bared. Acknowledging Jim Wilson as the source of the slide, Larry explains that the story of Dracula's death from a stake through the heart is clearly false, since the true cause was malnutrition.

"Huh?" arises from the audience.

"You can see that Dracula is standing behind the woman here, brandishing his teeth toward her posterior triangle, where no large blood vessels exist. He should be entering the anterior triangle, where the common carotid artery and the jugular vein are readily available." The students chuckle.

Up in the lab, the Team As are ready to present. They did the hand and now begin to crow that there is only one more dissection for this entire course. I hear more students talking about Thanksgiving and even Christmas vacations, plane tickets home and the like. As of today, nineteen dissection days have gone by, leaving eight to go, but these are some of the toughest dissections of all: the neck, the face, the eye, and other structures of the head. Although the hair of the cadavers has been clipped short to remove some of the "personal" signs, the head, like the pelvis, is one of the most value-laden areas of the body. No one directly says so, but the end of the course will have certain climactic drama.

I see more and more variation in anatomical methods now, as tables make up their own routines, often ignoring the *Dissector* and even the atlases. "Let's get this all skinned out for now," says Tim, undertaking the foot. "Then we can go home and read about what we should have been seeing." For many, the inductive approach (cut first, name later) seems to be the most effective. Tim, a former Broadway actor, likes direct, energetic approaches.

Greg takes me to his table in the next room, where Arnie has sawed the femur (thighbone) all the way through. He's cut muscles as well, so that the leg is completely detached and easy to manipulate. He says that the femur (the biggest bone of the body) took five or more minutes of concentrated sawing. We look at the severed semimembranosus muscle, one of the hamstrings. To our amazement, it is, on cross section, a thin shell of muscle surrounding a huge plug of fat. Absurdly enough, it looks like a fancy food preparation—a pastry, or a cheese-stuffed roll of meat.

"What the hell is this?" I ask.

"Makes no sense to us. Muscles aren't supposed to do that."

I ask a surgeon later that evening. He says it is extremely odd, perhaps a lipoma of some kind—a fat tumor. Every body in the lab seems to have its own oddities.

Back in the first room, a small assemblage of white-coated visitors walks around with a strange instrument, a tube with a long sensor. They are checking formaldehyde levels, as mandated by federal standards.

"Let's hold off on the rock," says Dr. English, pointing to a student radio just plugged in, turned up high. With the music off, the chatter and banter around the room also subsides. Eventually, the assessors leave.

"Who were *those* people?" Jonathan asks, recognizing the loss of good spirits in the room.

"Dr. English is not a fan of The Who," Steve observes. The students pass on the news that the formaldehyde levels were found to be acceptable—whatever that might mean. The sensor was placed right next to the cadaver to mimic the breathing of fumes by the dissectors, whose intent faces are often right next to body parts.

"That means we'll live long enough to repay our debts," one of them observes wryly. It's a joke of course, but it's also a recognition of some of the dangerous aspects of being a physician. Physicians often catch infections from patients (formerly—and now once again—tuberculosis, but also colds and hepatitis), suffer from depression, become impaired with alcohol and/or drugs, even commit suicide. One surgeon, infected with the HIV virus from a patient, has recently been in the news for suing the hospital where the transfer of the virus is alleged to have happened.

The formaldehyde assessors are the first of many "visitors" into the work of these future physicians: lawyers, insurors, hospital administrators; city, state, federal officials. Physicians have to deal with all of these pressures as well as our culture's impossible charge: *Save us from death and debility!*

A student pries loose a wad of fat, which flies onto her lip. She runs, in disgust, to the sink. Some weeks back, the story of such an event raised laughter as a distant absurdity. By now, something similar has probably happened to every one of the dissectors.

The radio is shortly back on, louder than before, belting out something that sounds to me like "Na nana na na nana na na na na." The students sing along, taking a cheerful revenge for the intrusion of the formaldehyde assessors. All med students and all physicians need to find their own Na NaNa Na Na to maintain their sanity, to avoid depression, to have the healing energy to pass on to a parade of depressed (and often depressing) patients. Many know how to do this well; I have seen and wondered at the apparently infinite good spirits of some plastic surgeons, for example, who reconstruct all kinds of ghastly injuries year round, year after year, meeting with patients, encouraging them, focusing on the healing ahead.

"I like classical music," Steve says, "but not while I'm cutting."

Conversation turns to a variety of foolish topics, and I spend the rest of my time working out seven-man touch football plays on three-by-five cards in response to a request from the med student football team. On such a tedious afternoon we all survive one way or another.

Having seen notice of a football game on the blackboard, I ask Steve, "Are you guys the Ovarian Cysters?"

"They are not," Kathy interrupts from the next table. "That is us, the girls' team, the Ovarian *Sisters*."

"Oh, of course. Well, what's the men's team?"

"The Sympathetic Chain Gang," Jonathan informs me—the pun relates to the sympathetic chain of nerves.

I recall Steve's earlier remark, "The jokes are one of the reasons you want to come up here."

We are finishing the eleventh week of a sixteen-week semester. Humor seems more important than ever for survival. These students have the heritage of Rabelais (a physician with gargantuan humor) and James Joyce (who had some medical training), who described the crude jokes of Buck Mulligan and his medical colleagues during the protracted labor of one Mrs. Mina Purefoy, in *Ulysses*. Even the term *humor* has a medical origin, the theory of the four humors that dominated Western medicine, from roots in the ancient Greece of Pythagoras to well into the Renaissance, roughly two thousand years. Bloodletting, for example, was considered an efficient means for removing an overabundance of blood, a tactic that was presumed to reduce fevers, but often resulted in the enfeeblement and death of a patient. This theory, corresponding to the four elements of earth, air, fire, and water, was slowly discredited as knowledge of the body became scientific, that is, scientific in the modern sense. In literature, a humor(ous) character is a person with a single humor (or basic fluid) that is so out of balance that he or she behaves in extreme fashion: a predominance of black bile gives you a melancholic or sad sack; a predominance of blood gives a sanguine or amorous character. Too much yellow bile creates the choleric or angry and impatient man. I'm quite sure there's a surplus of yellow bile on the interstate highways through and around Atlanta, especially at rush hour.

ONE DEGREE PER HOUR

· · ·

PAY A call on Jim Cooper, the embalmer. This is my first visit to the morgue, where he prepares the cadavers. Predictably, it is in the basement of the building—and unmarked. I try the handle. It is locked. I knock. He opens it. Two naked bodies lie on their backs on slanted tables. They are so obviously people, I am shocked.

One is an old man, with sprays of white hair. The other is a woman, with well-coiffed brown hair. They are naked, except for towels over their stomachs and genitals. The woman is tan; she is wearing fingernail polish. They are both a resounding pink, not gray. Their heads are propped up on little black stands. I gawk.

"Well, come on in!" Jim calls out cheerily. "I'm just getting these two finished up." Jim says it's unusual to have two at once—and he has been called to pick up another at a nearby hospital.

I watch him work over the next hour and ask him questions. He has already perfused these two corpses with formaldehyde, phenol, alcohol, and some pink dye, working through incisions in the neck and the groin. The added color gives a slightly aggressive pink to the flesh, which is certainly closer to life than the gray shades upstairs, but recognizable as somehow "not quite right." Jim sews up the four-inch incisions with cord. All of the blood has been displaced by the embalming fluid. This blood—some ten to fourteen pints per corpse—ran through a heavy tube directly into a drain in the floor.

"How does this whole process go?" I ask him.

"Well, first I wash the bodies and disinfect all the orifices." (The dead begin to deteriorate right away, once blood stops circulating; the bacteria in the bowel, for example, start to grow at a tremendous rate.) "Next, I make the incisions and get my fluid going. The easiest body to do is the perfectly healthy person who drops dead on the tennis court. I can do one of those with a neck incision only, since their circulatory system is so good. But that's a rarity. Many of our bodies come from nursing homes, and I'll need the groin incision also, perhaps even foot incisions as well."

"Where did you learn all this stuff?"

"You go to school. I used to work for a funeral home, but this is more interesting to me."

"What happens next?"

"After the perfusion, I ligate the cut arteries and veins and sew up the incision, like right now." Jim sews with a long, bent needle, something like an upholsterer's needle. He sews in quick, even stitches.

"When does the hair go?"

"I'll cut that off later on. This lady had hers done recently. A waste, as it turns out. She died of cancer—see the bronzing? We cut the hair off to depersonalize the body, to make it more of a generic corpse." I'm not really sure I can see the bronzing—maybe she is still a little orange? I forge ahead anyway.

"I've heard that hair and nails grow after death. Is that true?"

"No, it's not. Once the blood supply stops, all cells die. What does happen, though, is that the flesh shrinks due to the dehydration, and the nails and hair *appear* to grow, just from the withdrawal of the skin around them."

Jim is working with the woman's eyelids, trying to get them to lie down. "Right here, for example, she's drying out some, and the lids tend to open up." Her irises are blue. The pupils are huge black pools, "fixed and dilated," in the medical phrase.

"Edgar Allan Poe wrote something about premature burial," I say. "He describes a coffin with a lever system inside that could be used to raise a flag. You run into anything like that?"

"Well, not lately. There was much fascination with that in the nineteenth century and lots of techniques proposed. At one morgue, each station had a big ring to put over the cadaver's arm; then a string ran to a desk with a bell. If a patient wasn't really dead, the arm would move and the bell would ring."

"Was medicine so different that they could not tell if someone was dead?"

"No, but there were things they didn't understand, like cataleptic seizures that made people look dead. There were even coffins found with fingernail grooves on the inside of the lids, from persons who awakened after being buried."

"Ugh."

"Something like that happened to me once. I was treating a baby who had just died. I opened up the sternum to perfuse directly into the aorta and I saw that the heart was moving. If I was a cat, I'd say I lost about six of my nine lives right there."

"Jesus—what did you do?"

"I called the police for an escort and called the hospital and said, 'We're bringing this one back!' "

"What happened?"

"Well, the child really was dead, but the doctor said he had pumped a lot of Adrenalin into the heart, trying to get it going again. Apparently enough of the drug was still in the muscle to cause some of the fibers to contract—and that's what I saw."

I let all that sink in a while and watched him work. He is using a large syringe to inject embalming solution into the body cavities of the chest and abdomen. He pauses to check his work, then injects more into one of her thighs.

"How can you tell if she needs more?"

"By feel. Get some gloves." Jim pulls open a cabinet door, and I take one left and one right glove from two boxes.

"Now feel right here, how good and stiff it is."

I feel. It feels solid. And not warm.

"Now over here, how loose it is."

Well, of course it is, I think. *That's the inside of her thigh.* I feel. It is malleable, the way a woman's inner thigh should be—but cold.

"Of course she has more fat there," he says, injecting more solution into the area. Evidently he can correlate body turgidity with the proper amount of chemicals.

"How fast does a body lose heat?" I ask him.

"Well, the medical examiner figures one degree per hour, very roughly speaking, and that's Fahrenheit. There are all kinds of factors, like the weather or air conditioning or blankets, but for a rough rule of thumb that'll do. So when the M.E. sets a time of death, it's usually by the rectal temperature. If it's ninety-two degrees, the person died about six hours ago. Of course, you get some exceptions. We had one corpse that measured out at a hundred and six degrees, eight hours later. The M.E. said, 'That's got to be meningitis,' and he put all of us who had anything to do with the case on drugs. The temperature always goes up a little bit initially anyway, as some metabolic activity continues in the body but the blood no longer takes away the heat. Then the temperature falls."

(I learn later that this rule of thumb is so approximate that some physicians consider it useless; many detective writers, however, like its terseness and routinely put it into their stories.)

"What's in all those bags?" There are about ninety brown paper bags lined up on wooden shelves, each neatly numbered.

"That's cremated remains. We store them there until they are claimed or buried."

"How come they are such different sizes?" Some are like a loaf of bread, while others are double that.

"Well, it's like different people are different sizes. This man here is a lot bigger than this lady." He nods to the two corpses between us. "The cremation burns up all the fat, muscle, tendons, and the like, so all you really have left is the bones. Then those are ground up and put in a bag. A big man or woman gives you lots of leftover bones. A little woman with osteoporosis gives you a small amount."

Jim finishes up his work and says, "Well, I need to pick up a body. Do you want to come along?"

Shortly we are riding in a white "hearse," but it looks more like a cross between a panel truck and a station wagon. I have walked past this vehicle in the parking lot a hundred times without giving it a thought. (The big, fancy black hearses that funeral homes use can cost $60,000, certainly out of a university's price range.)

At the hospital Jim removes the folding gurney from the back, and we go to an office to do the paperwork. Then to the hospital morgue—unmarked—where the body lies in a cooler. Compared to the corpses I've been seeing, it's a relatively young man, perhaps in his fifties, with a barrel chest.

"That's a big one," Jim says, just looking at the plastic covering. "Perhaps near our limit of two hundred and fifty pounds." He transfers the covered body from one stretcher to the other, feet first, then hips, then chest.

"Okay, let's wash our hands again."

Soon we are riding back to the anatomy building. Jim backs the vehicle down a ramp I have walked by often but never really seen. Now I know that directly behind that wall Jim works his craft on 200 bodies a year. The quality of his work is crucial to the work of Cliff and David, Jonathan and Steve, Jocelyn and Lisa, and all of the other students upstairs, this year, and every year.

Later in the year, Jim takes me on a visit to a funeral home with a crematorium. The funeral director says that the burning gas reaches 2,000°F, hot enough to consume bodies in two or three hours. He explains that the limbs burn first, entirely, then the head—burning completely—while the torso, being thicker, requires more time. Most of the body, therefore, actually goes up the chimney as steam and gases. The eventual remains are chunks of the heaviest and best-protected bones, the lower vertebrae and pelvis. These fragments are swept up from the oven and put into a processor, which can reduce them to almond-sized bits, or to flakes, or even to sand, depending on the machine and its setting. The director shows me a can of bone flakes, and I stir my finger in them. They feel like surf-beaten bits of shell or fine china.

They are light in color, about what you'd expect bone fragments to be, not at all charred. Nonetheless, we call them "the ashes" of the body. I'm glad to see these fragments finally and to assess what they mean to me: they seem mundane, common, even trivial. I don't know what choices my mother was offered regarding the final disposition of my father's ashes, and I have occasionally wondered whether we should have done more for his remains. Seeing these little bits of bone tells me that they weren't worth such trouble—at least according to my values. I respect nonetheless the choices other families have made to save the ashes or to scatter them in places important to the dead person.

(Not long after writing these words, I participated in the burial of my father-in-law, Harvey F. Corson. After the church service, family members went to the graveside, where a handsome wooden chest held the ashes from his cremation. We laid roses by his chest and some of us touched it to bid farewell once last time. For all of us, these were symbols that gave closure and healing.)

A PRETTY COOL PERSON

· · ·

THE DISSECTORS HAVE been working their way down the body, from the torso, through the pelvis and upper leg—with a detour for the arm—to the lower leg and foot. The cadavers are pretty well cut up now (except for the head) so that the students comment on the difficulty of turning the body over, with all the scraps and tatters. "It weighs a lot less now," one student says, "but it's harder to keep it all together." For the most part students now say "it," not "him" or "her." Today, however, the working "down the body" will end. Team B—Steve and Jonathan—must present the calf and foot, but Team C—Lisa and Jocelyne—will head upward to the neck, the first of four dissections on the head.

"The goddamn head's going to be something else," one student says as we go up the stairs. We have just seen a lecture on the eye by a surgeon who repairs eye injuries. His slides—of injuries and operations—were startling, arresting, even disturbing. One series of slides showed a stab wound to the eye, which left a big chunk of the knife blade broken off—and hidden in the eye—for months, so that the metal actually began to rust. Somehow several physicians and hospitals failed to diagnose the obvious cause of this patient's headaches. "Always get an X ray!" the lecturer proclaimed.

Another series showed the process of taking out an eyeball and putting in a prosthesis (an artificial eye) with the muscles reattached, so that a false eye would move parallel to the remaining healthy eye. Afterward, one student tells me he was shaking all over during that part of the lecture. Another says he was getting so upset he almost left the room.

Even while Steve and Jonathan work on their presentation, Lisa starts to skin the back of the neck of the cadaver. The centenarian lies facedown, her head, for once, completely uncovered. She has some wisps of white hair on the back of her head; otherwise, the hair has been clipped very close. Lisa strokes the hair with her hand, then focuses on the thin, wrinkled neck.

Steve and Jonathan are concerned about the time for their presentation: they are over the ten-minute limit. During the next hour, they go through it five times, talking faster and cutting the length, until it fits. Gail and Maggie are among the early listeners, following the details of bones, muscles, vasculature, and the like. They smile when Steve shows the action of the bones: he has detached the lower leg and foot from the articulated skeleton and moves these bones to illustrate flexion, rotation, and pronation. The bare bones dance between the lamp and the cadaver on the table. I think of the danse macabre of Halloween a few weeks ago, but this reanimation dance is not only bony but cheerful.

It is generally known that John and Larry, at Table 1, have something special planned for the end of their presentation, so the room gets very quiet as they reach the end of their ten minutes.

"And so, Dr. Wolf, we end our presentation, hoping that we didn't put our foot in our mouth this time." One student brings the skeletal foot toward his mouth and the other brings the cadaver's foot (nearly sawn off) toward his mouth. There is a quiet laughter around the room except for Steve, who laughs heartily—*brays,* one might say—from Table 3; some students stare at him, as he continues to laugh. Dr. Wolf shakes his head at this cheerful lunacy and asks some questions about the dissection.

Shortly Steve and Jonathan give their version formally and finish in nine minutes thirty seconds.

Dr. Wolf twits them, "You have a whole half a minute left!"

Steve: "That's because we wanted you to have plenty of time for questions." (The whole room is listening to this exchange.)

Dr. Wolf: "Okay, do you play sports?"

Steve: "Not professionally."

Dr. Wolf: "What are the deltoid ligaments?"

Steve: "They are right here." He points them out.

Dr. Wolf: "Good, and how about the spring ligaments?"

Steve: "Right here," again locating them.

Dr. Wolf: "Right again, and if you sprain your foot playing basketball, in an eversion sprain, that's what you'll probably tear."

Steve: "Michigan is number three right now."

Dr. Wolf: "Tell that to someone who cares."

They all laugh. Dr. Wolf takes them into the hall for their feedback and grade.

Returning to the room, Jonathan congratulates Steve on knowing those names, adding "You goober, I thought we were really *going to get it* with that 'extra time for questions'!"

Lisa has been cutting away on the back of the neck all the while, skinning and picking fat. The men help her turn the body over, and Steve takes particular care to wet down the legs and cover them with paper towels. The men depart, and Lisa works steadily away at the front of the neck.

The old woman's face is up now, and uncovered. Her eyes are shut, her toothless mouth hangs open. Her tongue is the same grayish pink as the rest of her face. Her cheeks have two yellow spots over the cheekbones, where the skin has become translucent from drying out and the fat below shows through. It is certainly an old face, with wrinkles and "age spots," although it seems to me that the wrinkles may have been plumped back out somewhat by the embalming. Suddenly Lisa says, "She must have been a pretty cool person to give her body for this." I like her formulation a lot, since it represents a relationship between not only the living and the dead but between the generations.

The neck is tricky, since important nerves are just under the skin, and many important structures in the front are closely packed. At a neighboring table, Karl points out the platysma, a thin muscle covering the front of the neck, that his partner Charlie has carefully dissected free of the skin of the Fatless Man. Later Charlie mentions Karl's Law: "The human body is primarily made up of fat and connective tissue; all other parts are incidental." This sentiment is verbal vengeance on the considerable fat-picking necessary on all these bodies, even the Fatless Man.

Several of the cadavers have their mouths open, as if some song might rise from their gray lips. At some tables, the thin flaps of the neck skin and platysma are pulled up and stuck into the mouth, to keep them out of the way. This sight is arresting at first, but it makes a lot of practical sense. Certainly any notion of the cadavers eating themselves is absurd, but an even more bizarre and suggestive notion comes to mind: I think of the medieval paintings showing persons speaking in scrolls of words that issue from their mouths; perhaps, symbolically, the cadavers are singing themselves into focus, into being. In death, the song of the cadaver is its own material, the melody is one more gift, a concert of flesh for these students to hear.

SAY IT TO HIS FACE

• • •

T'S CHILLY AND windy this November day. Most of the leaves have blown out of the trees, leaving them skeletal against gray skies. Underfoot, the leaves rapidly lose color and shape. I think of the skin, fat, and muscles falling off the cadavers, leaving the basic structure behind, not all the way down to the skeleton, usually, but certainly deeper into a person than we ordinarily see. The forthcoming dissections of the head will get us closer to the bone than in most of the previous dissections. Somehow, we shall be entering the skull.

The students are counting down the labs on their way to Christmas: each team has only one more dissection to do. But there is apprehension in the air, much like the nervousness about dissecting the pelvis. We have three dissections of the head to go, including the face, the eye, and the removal of the brain. There is a rumor that the head itself is to be cut entirely away from the body. I ask one student whether there is more curiosity or dread regarding the dissection of the head.

"Dread—hands down," he replies.

Although the students talk about their fears in general terms, they aren't very specific about what will happen. The cuts are specified in their syllabi, generally close at hand; apparently the students are choosing *not* to know the details. Instead, they speculate on how the cuts will go—around the head, like a hat brim, or straight through from the front, splitting the chin, nose, and forehead. For each suggestion, they gesture with their hands around their own heads, rather an eerie symbol—as if their own heads were going to be dismantled, as if their hands were like magic wands that could divide flesh and bone.

Even with the neck, I feel we are closer to the humanity of these cadavers than ever before: they lie on their backs, with heads raised by one or even two wooden blocks. They look like people in bed propped up to read. The white plastic and blanket covers them from the chest on down, with the feet well tucked in. In a sense, the rest of the body is finished, from here to the end, it's the head only. (The last lab will bring the foot back into view, but, for now, the rest of the body is covered and forgotten.)

We can't pretend that these corpses are fetal pigs or sharks: the actual faces are entirely bare and raised into prominence. As the students bend over them, the cadavers' heads and the students' are on the same level, inches apart, as if they were equals in intimate conversation. At all tables the lamps are set to illumine the neck and, spilling upward, the light shines on the students' faces as well. The students now use their lamps effectively; all faces, dead and alive, look like they are spotlighted on stage.

The cadaveric faces are all different from each other, presumably as they were in life. Heavier male features—nose, jaw, ridge over the eyes—stand out from the lighter female features. All eyes are either closed or slitted. Students look into the eye now and then, pulling the lid back with a gloved finger. Most are fogged and somewhat slack, but recognizably eyes. (Some of the corneas have been harvested for transplantation; this is the only tissue from an old person that will work well when transplanted.) None of these eyes have much to say, although the students seem to want to know whether any messages might be there. After looking within and finding little, they push the lids shut.

One man describes being up in the lab last Saturday night. "It was dark, of course, and several of us were here, but about midnight, I realized that everyone had left except me, and the eyelid on my specimen was slowly raising and that he was *looking at me.* I thought *Well, this is ridiculous; he can't really see anything,* but it seemed eerie, so I closed the eye—two or three times, until it stayed shut."

"That would have *freaked me out,*" one woman comments, rolling her eyes.

Despite the differences in the cadavers, some features are common. Noses are bent to the side, because of the bending of cartilage under pressure of the head when the cadaver lay facedown. Some lips are flattened as well. Many cadavers now have yellow spots on the cheekbones. At Table 2, Fred looks determined, focused. At Table 1, Rose looks frail, ancient. At Table 6, Quasi is delicate. At Table 5, Nero is powerful, robust; even his platysma muscles are large. Conversation continues on his size, once again, in the usual ritual. Two students are joking about him at the far end of the room when Alex, cutting on Nero, suddenly says, "If you want to say anything about Nero, say it to his face." The joking stops, and conversation takes another direction.

Was Alex just bantering, or was he serious? Was he protecting Nero from gossip, protecting his anatomical "partner"? Now that the faces are, indeed, bare, there is a power of the person—or the past person—that is stronger than ever before. This new humanization will make the head dissection even more difficult.

Because the necks are stretched, the mouths now hang open. Bending over the neck, students appear to be turning an ear to these cadaveric mouths, as if to catch any last words.

Lisa and Jocelyne are trying to match words and structures, quite a job today. With the limbs, structures were spread out and clear; in the neck, the nerves are all jammed together with blood vessels in a tangle that becomes worse as structures are dissected free. At a neighboring table I hear, "Let's try to name these things." At another table, "What is this damn stuff?" At another, "Look at all these dumb little strings!" (I think of "dumb" in its other meaning of "nonspeaking" and recall student requests that body parts somehow talk.) Further complicating matters, there is considerable individual variation in the neck; for example, nerves and blood vessels can supply a given muscle from above or below.

It's a searching-and-naming day, with constant reference to the atlases or instructors, who must, themselves, trace back structures to larger structures or bony landmarks to find their way. The neck is a tangle, everyone agrees, and work proceeds very slowly, tediously, in this room and in all the others. I am bored and take a trip to Room 2.

In the next room, the blackboard is full of writing.

ON THE BLACKBOARD OF ROOM 2

(Figure 23)

Oh	Our	On	Olfactory	Some
Oh	Old	Old	Optic	Say
Oh	Oak	Olympus	Oculomotor	Marilyn
To	Tree	Towering	Trochlear	Monroe's
Try	Takes	Tops	Trigeminal	But
And	Away	A	Abducens	My
Find	Fresh	Finn	Facial	Brother
A	Air	And	Auditory	Says
Good	Giving	German	Glossopharyngeal	Brigitte
Vaccine	Very	Vend	Vagus	Bardot's are
Striking	Shady	Some	Spinal Accessory	More
Herpes	Homes	Hops	Hypoglossal	Massive

Column three ("On Old Olympus") looks familiar, since it is the traditional mnemonic for the twelve cranial nerves (whose anatomic names are shown in column four). But what are these others? I ask around and learn that David (Thies), at a neighboring table, has put out calls for new versions, which students have provided in the first two columns. The fifth (last) column is witty in its rhyme and possessives but impenetrable to me; I feel like a patient confronted with incomprehensible jargon.

"So what's the deal with Monroe and Bardot?" I ask.

"We felt we should have a device for remembering which nerves are sensory, which were motor, and which are both," David explains. Suddenly S, M, and B, as initials, makes sense. I wish medical explanations to patients could always be so clear.

I stop at the table of Lisa (Drake) and Gail, who are using their color-coded system once again. The neck bristles with string and heads of pins. I ask them about the removal of the top of the head.

"Just saw right around," one of them says.

"With what—a power saw?" I have seen this done in the autopsy room; it goes fairly quickly.

"Nope. With that." They indicate a plain handsaw, about ten inches long. "And the trick will be not to damage the contents within by breaking through too quickly!" Although I can't imagine doing it that way, the prospect of this task doesn't seem to daunt them at all.

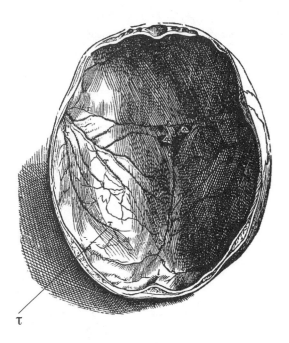

τ

THE TOP OF THE SKULL

(Figure 24)

From *De fabrica,* page 24.

IF THE TOP of the skull is set on a table, it looks like this. The lines inside
are either sutures where bones join (the straighter lines meeting in a right
angle) or curving grooves corresponding to the blood vessels of the meninges
(coverings of the brain; here labeled with the Greek letter tau—"τ").

The front of the head is here uppermost, with holes in the bone that are
portions of the frontal sinuses.

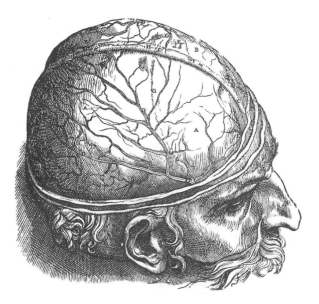

THE BRAIN IN THE SKULL

(Figure 25)

From *De fabrica,* page 606.

TODAY'S DISSECTORS MAKE the same "hat brim" cut around the skull to allow for removing the top of the skull.

"C," on the forehead, indicates the falx cerebri dividing the two halves of the cerebral cortex, or neocortex (new brain). "D" marks a blood vessel in the dura ("A"). Each convolution or curl of brain tissue is technically known as a gyrus; each corresponding groove is a sulcus.

The mustache and beard, partially visible, remind us of the cadaver's past humanity.

YOU'RE HOLDING A LIFE
IN YOUR HAND
· · ·

ODAY'S THE DAY: we embark upon the head. Twice I have heard students discuss the possibility of the heads actually exploding when the skull is penetrated. In one discussion, a student pooh-poohed the possibility: "Even if there's considerable pressure, the first few cuts through the bone would relieve it, like, you know, the valve on a pressure cooker." The other students considered this surreal image and dropped the subject. I have heard an instructor say that brains are one of the hardest areas to embalm properly and that, some years, a few of the brains have started to decay by the end of the course. This year's embalming seems, however, to have done the job well.

"X marks the spot!" David says cheerfully, as he and Cliff start to peel the skin on the top of their cadaver's skull. One cut goes from her forehead over the top of her head, while the other cut goes from ear to ear, again over the top. The resulting X gives four corners to peel back, and soon all six Team As are making quick progress, even before the Team Cs have begun to present the dissection of the neck. There are several reasons for the students' alacrity with this cutting. It's a complicated dissection, with lots of steps, including opening the top of the head and removing the brain—as well as dissecting the face and the eye. Some of these students are going home for Thanksgiving but must present on the following Tuesday. This is the last dissection of the course for Team A. Last, there is considerable inherent interest in this area. Jonathan, for example, is touring necks today, but he is eager to see the brain.

"I can't wait for them to get the head open. This is one of the most interesting areas!" he says.

There is some predictable discussion about scalping, and the notion that a person could survive being scalped if the skin could grow back over the pericranium, the layer of tissue over the skull.

"And what did the ancients do, boring those little holes?" one student calls out.

"Trepanation . . . to let the bad spirits out," is the answer from another table. "There are neolithic skulls with those holes healed over, suggesting that some people actually survived the operation."

"Yeah, and some of the holes weren't little at all," another adds. "I've seen pictures: they were more like this." She holds up the circle of her thumb and forefinger joined. Some of us give a little shiver. After surgery to remove cancerous tissue, my dad had a fist-sized hole in his skull. A nurse who came to watch him during the night asked on her first visit, "Does he have a window? You always have to be careful of that."

Steve is unexpectedly dressed up today: a nice pink shirt, a tie, and a white lab jacket.

"What's the deal?" his classmates ask him, pulling his tie out of his buttoned jacket and stuffing the ends in the breastpocket. They turn up the back of his jacket collar in a style once implying juvenile delinquency. These gestures suggest familiarity on the one hand, but perhaps also criticism: is Steve a turncoat, appearing to be a real doctor instead of a student in T-shirt and jeans? Symbolically, he is a traitor, "dressed for success," in an advertising slogan of the 1980s. At some level, none of the students are eager to deliver medical care quite yet; why should Steve appear to be?

"I've got to go visit a patient for one of my classes. He's got a terminal disease," Steve says seriously, readjusting his clothes—without playing along with the jokes. "I saw him some weeks back, and it was real depressing. He can hardly do anything because of a lung disease. I'm going to see him today and see if he's feeling any better—even though he can't get well."

Several of us fall into a conversation about the healing role of a physician beyond the medical response. Steve says, "One of the things I learned talking to him was that it might be hard to do both at once—relate to him as a person and still come up with the right medical analysis."

"Yeah, but that's really the thing," Larry says, "because your patients want to believe in what you're doing, and if you talk to them about medicine only, they may just blow you off."

From the patient's point of view, belief in the healing power of the physician comes from the obvious technical knowledge, as well as from the physician's signs and words of caring. In his book *A Leg to Stand On,* Oliver Sacks (a physician himself) describes his disappointment when, as a patient, he can't get the humane attention of his surgeon.

This noon is the second meeting to plan the Service of Reflection and Gratitude; students report on their various committees, the performers, the refreshments. As we break up, a woman asks Don whether he'd be up in the lab this afternoon. "Yes, I'll be up there," he said.

"Good," she said, "because the next team is going to cut into her face. This is the last time Agnes will be recognizable as Agnes. Once her face is gone—that's it!"

Lisa and Jocelyne are fixing up the last details of the neck and running over their presentation. They have done a fine job on this complicated area, separating and labeling the mass of nerves, arteries, veins, and small muscles. They ask me to time their presentation, which lasts nine minutes and fifty-two seconds. "Wow, eight whole seconds to spare!" they crow.

The Team As start to work around the Team Cs. They peel the skin back on the skull, so that the six heads in the room look like flowers of flesh, the large bulge of each calvaria appearing amidst the four pointed flaps of the scalp peeling outward. (*Calvarium* is the root for "Calvary," meaning "Golgotha"—the place of the skull.) The scalp peels back readily, and there is little beneath to be careful about, some muscle fibers, a little fat in some cases, but mostly the periosteum directly covering the bones of the skull. At one table, students rip the skin back by hand.

There is a renewed discussion of the "head box" in the next room, where various heads and necks float in preservative fluid. At our table, we discuss the paradox of how grisly the sight of these random heads is, but how everyone wants to see anyway. It is a good theme for the day, since the medical students simultaneously dread the dissection of the head and feel great curiosity about it.

The students discuss a rumor that the lab instructors will actually do the cutting of the skulls, and, before long, there is verification. Dr. Rizzolo asks for attention and says, "We want to open all the heads today. I need bare bone, clean and dry, in a plane like this." He gestures around his own head at the level where a man's hat brim would rest. Cliff and David have the skull's skin all pulled back and have moved on to the face, peeling the skin off the cheeks, which are full of golden fat. They have cut around the eyes and the mouth, leaving three ghostly circles, while all the rest of the skin comes off. As opposed to the thick, tough skin over the skull, the skin on the cheeks and nose is paper thin.

"Boy, we'd better get this periosteum off of the skull," one of them says, since they are eager to get the brain out today.

Jonathan beckons to me from the door, and I follow him into the next room. Dr. Rizzolo is carrying a cast saw, an electric hand tool covered in shiny stainless steel, ending in a small half-moon blade. This blade vibrates in plaster or bone, tearing it apart, with minimal risk to the soft tissues underneath (although it can raise a patient's anxiety to astronomic heights, as anyone who has been through this experience well knows). Rizzolo looks at several skulls to see whether they are ready for his machine. Jonathan follows him eagerly. No skulls are ready in this room, so we go back to the first room.

Rizzolo likes what he sees at Table 1, so he hands the saw's electric cord to a student to plug it in. Rizzolo places the short, curved blade on the cadaver's bony forehead and throws the switch. The saw is loud—whining and snarling—as the blade vibrates and cuts. Plumes of thin smoke arise, and students wrinkle their noses against the smell of burning bone and make com-

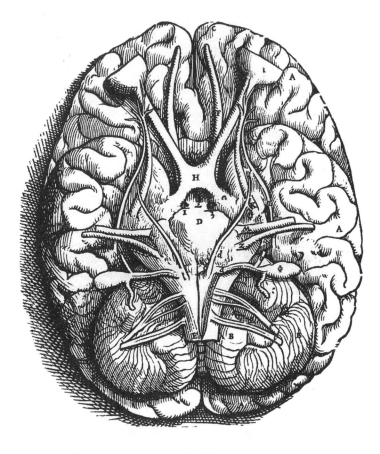

The Base of the Brain

(Figure 26)

From *De fabrica*, page 318.

ROLLED OUT OF the skull, the brain comes out in one piece, if the spinal cord ("E") is cut. The cranial nerves tear, however, often at the point where they enter holes (foramina) in the base of the skull.

According to Saunders and O'Malley, Vesalius (and Galen) understood seven pairs of nerves (not the modern twelve), and did not include the olfactory nerves ("F") in their count.

The optic nerves ("I") cross at their chiasma ("H"). Others, visible as stalks, are interpreted differently today.

The cerebellum, the "old brain," tightly coiled, is labeled "B".

The cerebrum, much larger, is the modern brain, also known as the "neo-cortex," marked three times with the letter "A."

Although Vesalius didn't understand the brain very well by modern standards, this illustration gives a good idea of the clarity of the cranial nerves at the base of the brain.

ments about a dentist's office. A dozen students crowd around the end of the table to see this extraordinary event.

"Oh shit," someone says.

The sight is arresting: Rizzolo makes his way around one side of the head, then the other, with slow, steady progress. The dozen students crowd around, craning their necks to see. After two minutes of sawing, Rizzolo takes a probe to test whether the cut is through; he finds one intact section, saws that free, then lifts the top of the skull off. The free piece of bone looks like the upper shell of a turtle, but uniform in color. Rizzolo places it upside down on the table, where it rests like an oval, shallow bowl. Everyone strains to see the exposed brain. (See Figures 24 and 25 above.)

Rizzolo uses a scalpel to cut through the dura mater, the outermost layer of tissue protecting the brain, and explains the terms for the various folds as they come into our view. The uppermost fold, the falx cerebri (the "sickle of the two halves of the neocortex") divides the brain vertically, from front to back, creating a groove, called the superior saggital sinus, a venous lake that gathers blood from the brain and sends it downward through an ingenious drainage system to, finally, the jugular vein. With the dura mater (literally the "tough mother") out of the way, he works more deeply, to remove the brain from the skull. With its two lobes of twisting patterns, the brain looks much like the twin halves of an elaborate walnut, still partially in its shell. The nut of the brain "sprouts" downward into the spinal cord, which, in turn, branches throughout the body.

With a scalpel he separates the brain from attachments on the sides and bottom and, finally, severs the spinal cord itself at the base of the brain. He rolls the brain out of the head toward himself, bringing the cerebellum and the pons along with the cerebral cortex. All of us watching are mesmerized.

Dr. Rizzolo holds the brain upside down and shows the severed cranial nerves as they sprout from its base. (See Figure 26 above.) "Here's the olfactory bulbs, the optic chiasma, here's the oculomotor, this would be the trochlear, and here's the trigeminal. . . ." (On the board behind him is yet one more mnemonic for these twelve nerves: "Oh, Oh, Oh, To Touch And Find A Girl's Vagina, Ah, Heaven," the "Ah" standing for Spinal Accessory;

this formulation goes well back in time, when women in medical school were a rarity.) He shows the students the Circle of Willis (the loop of arteries at the base of the brain). He points inside the skull and shows where nerves and blood vessels go through the floor of the skull. Everyone around the table gawks and cranes to see these strange sights.

Dr. Rizzolo moves on to open another skull, and Pete and Bill look at the newly opened body parts. "This is incredible," Pete says, "it's all here, just like it should be." After the crowded complexity of the neck, the brain seems not only dramatic, but clear. Pete and Bill show the cranial nerves to other students who drop by to see this first of nineteen heads to be opened today. Pete hefts the brain in his gloved hand. "It weighs a little something," he says. "And to think that you're holding someone's life in your hand, all the memories, everything," he says in awe.

"She'll never miss it now," Bill says.

"True enough. But this is where she was aware of herself," Pete continues, pointing to the frontal lobe. All of us around the table take in his comment with our own brains, similarly shaped, but softer without embalming, and, of course, *alive*.

We look inside the head, an irregular but symmetrical cup lined with more dura. No one has had this view of this particular head before. The remaining folds of the dura are a shiny gray, with iridescent highlights. We can see the horizontal folds of the dura called the tentorium; this structure supports the neocortex and divides it from the lower cerebellum and the brain stem. Bill and Pete find the foramina (holes) through which the cranial nerves run; they locate the vertebral arteries coming through the foramen magnum, the large hole where the spinal cord exits the skull. The actual cord looks like a whitish rope, about the thickness of a thumb.

Other students come by and look in. *Amazing* and *incredible* are the two most common responses.

After the crowd thins, I take a look and ask to hold the brain. I put a few paper towels on my hand and Pete lowers the brain onto them.

"It's heavy," he says.

Since he lowers the brain upside down into my hand, its curved upper surface fits my palm well, much like the heart Karl shared with me weeks ago, but this is much denser, heavier. It feels like a big bag of water, but represents one of the clearest differences between human beings and all the other animals. I look at this strange thing in my hand, truly an improbable object. And yet this is the primary organ I try to reach in my students and readers. Now a brain has, in a sense, reached me. What does it have to say to me, heavy and sodden, its many curves shining in the bright light? I think of the gross insult to my father, a man of intellect: brain cancer. Aha, maybe this was his revenge: teaching with his brain even past illness and death.

This brain is now dead matter, primarily fat and water—material that will eventually burn so completely as to leave no ash at all. This brain functions now, however, as a catalytic mirror, as we respond to it anatomically or associationally. This inelegant mass makes it possible for us to read, hear music, sense pleasure, and experience our deepest loves. In many ways it represents the central definition of what it is to be human.

I return to Table 3, where Rizzolo has just opened the head of the centenarian. Her brain comes out easily, leaving the dural fold pretty much intact within her skull. These folds provide an elegant system of three-dimensional shock absorbency for the brain, which is relatively delicate. Brain tissue has within it no bone, no tendon, no ligament; it has a large fat component (all the lipid coverings of neurons): if anyone calls you "fathead," you can justifiably reply, "That's correct," and/or "Thank you." In life, the tissue is less dense and more like jelly, easily injured by a blow or compression through bleeding within the rigid skull.

Cliff and David make their survey of the severed cranial nerves on the bottom of the brain and show me the structures of the floor of the skull. But there is other work for today, and they put the brain away in a Tupperware container and turn, again, to the face.

I'LL NEVER DO THIS AGAIN

• • •

HAVE YOU SEEN what's going on up there?" several students ask me. "They're taking off the tops of the heads!" They are abuzz about the lab, whether they are part of the current dissection or not, since students who aren't cutting have dropped by to witness the dramatic event. The cutting, they say, went until 6:00 P.M., when all nineteen were finished. "By the end, Dr. Rizzolo had little fragments of bone and cadaver juice all over his glasses," one says.

I stop by the lab Friday afternoon, and see a half a dozen teams working hard now to have their Thanksgiving time unencumbered. Several of them have cut down the frontal bone over the eye, from the hairline to the eye socket, but David and Cliff have found everything they want from the inside of the skull, working out toward the eye, leaving the bone of the forehead intact.

"How'd you do that?" I ask them, looking at their handiwork.

"The old hammer and chisel," they report, although they also say that the frontal bone that covers the top of the eye was paper thin, delicate enough to pierce with a pair of forceps.

They are happy today. Their dissection is a success. And, to top it off, they have big news: "We beat the Ambulance Chasers—the better law school team—by thirteen to zip!" This is a modern Holy War, lawyers versus doctors, two professions with high motivations, high ideals, and many competitive personalities. Lawyer jokes have been making the rounds in the lab: "What do you call twenty lawyers at the bottom of the ocean?" "A good start." And: "What's the difference between a dead possum and a dead lawyer on the highway?" "The possum has skid marks in front of it."

Saturday afternoon, David and Cliff are the only ones in the lab. When I arrive, David is sitting on a stool at the end of the table, peering into the open skull of their cadaver, whose head, face up, is propped up on two layers of wooden block. Cliff is behind him, looking over his shoulder; a light is behind Cliff, shining directly into the skull. The large round lampshade and the smaller, cuplike skull form parentheses around the intact spheres of the two men's heads.

"Hey, come see all the stuff we've found," they call out excitedly. I grab a lab coat and join them. They show me the foramina (holes in the base of the skull) and the various nerves and blood vessels, including the sinus cavernosus, a kind of gathering pool for venous blood, just before it enters the internal jugular vein. They poke at the tissues carefully, sometimes warning each other, "Don't tear it off! It's fragile!"

They show me the hypophyseal fossa (also known as the Turkish saddle, or sella turcica), where the all-important pituitary gland lies. A fragment of its stalk sticks up, torn off when the brain came out. Deep in the base of the skull, the pituitary gland, the "master gland," is extraordinarily well protected. Surgery on it is difficult; sometimes the approach must be up through the nose.

"We gotta sprinkle all this," Cliff says, shaking the preserving-fluid bottle. "If you don't keep the nerves wet, they dry out and turn yellow. And *break*." He gives a shudder worthy of a seasoned dissector.

Cliff takes his turn at the head of the table, while David searches in the manuals and syllabi.

"Oh wow, check this out," Cliff calls out. "The nasal ciliary nerve goes through the muscle here . . . no, wait, just under it. . . ." He tugs gently at an air sac, and pulls it out. "Great!" he cries. "This is part of the ethmoid sinus, one of the air cells," he says, holding up a small, semitransparent, irregular sac. "When your sinuses fill up or get infected, it's one of these jobs." The sacs provide mucus to help wash through the nasal areas, but they also relieve the weight of the head. Solid bone would require even more muscular and skeletal support.

"Did you get a good look at a brain yet?" David asks me. David takes the brain out of a large Tupperware container, where it floats in preservative fluid. The ancient cerebellum (at the lower back of the brain) looks like a small bundle of tan, parallel cords. Above it, the larger cerebrum—the modern brain—has thin ropes in the wonderful twisting pattern of gyrus and sulcus (turn and groove). David turns the brain over and he and Cliff trace the twelve cranial nerves and the blood supply for me.

The olfactory bulbs (by which we can interpret smells) lie on the front of the base of the brain and extend forward, looking like antennae.

"Look here," David says, pointing within the skull, and he shows me the ethmoid (sieve-shaped) bone near the midline of the skull. "We've destroyed one side, but here, just by the crista galli [cock's comb] you can see the groove where the olfactory bulb lies on top and extends nerve fibers into the top of the nasal area. This is called the cribriform plate." (*Cribriform* is the literal Latin equivalent of the Greek *ethmoid,* both meaning "sieve-shaped.") It is through this intricate arrangement that the smells of turkey stuffing and gravy will reach our consciousness next week on Thanksgiving Day.

"And you've got to see the face," Cliff says, pulling the blanket down. The cadaver is still recognizably the same individual, even though skin and fat are dissected away, leaving three circles of normal skin at the mouth and the eyes. Oddly enough, she looks for a brief instant like a young girl, say fourteen years old, with thin cheeks, but full lips. Cliff shows me the muscles of the jaw and lips, including the superficial muscles of the face that, under the fat layer, give the face expression. Here's the parotid duct, bringing saliva from the parotid gland in front of the ear to an opening high in the mouth. Cliff says, "You can feel that duct, running horizontally, if you clench your jaw muscle [masseter] and stroke up and down over it, so that you 'roll' the duct." He strokes his cheek; I stroke mine. Yes, there it is, small but distinct.

Cliff is poking inside the skull again. "I'll never do this again in my life," he says quietly.

SHE GAVE HER BEST

. . .

HERE'S NO LECTURE today, so I head up to the lab about one-thirty. Only a dozen students are scattered through the rooms. We are closing in on the Thanksgiving holiday, and some students have already left the campus. The drama of dissecting the head continues, nonetheless, and some students are talking about the dissection for the next week, when the head, according to the syllabus, will be sawn in half.

Jackie LaPorte and Jim Newsom, the lab coordinators, seem to have some latitude to talk to me, so I ask them about the Tupperware containers for the brains.

"Do you mean the canisters or the cake-takers?" Jackie asks me. I'm not sure, especially since I've never heard the phrase "cake-taker," which I guess to be "cake-bell" in my dialect or "cake-saver" in my wife's.

"If you mean the containers for the brains, we use the cake-takers for those, since they'll hold an entire brain and another half a brain, plus your liquid, of course. The students just take the brain out in the fall; they'll need it again for the Neuro course in the spring," Jackie explains. "The plastic containers in there now are regular old canisters, like for sugar or flour, you know." Jim says that these hold six quarts. "We've had some of them in use for thirty years," he adds.

I ask Jim, who is double-wrapping human-tissue refuse from the labs (scraps of skin and fat, typically), where that stuff will be going.

"To the crematory," he says, indicating the eventual destination for all of the cadavers.

"I'll show you something, if you want," Jackie says, and takes me to some cabinets in one of the labs. I look up at the shelves, not sure of what I'm seeing: stacks of square plastic trays with notations like *Torso, 3* and *Leg, 6*.

"What is this?" I ask.

"Why, these are cross sections. You know"—she cuts her hand along her waist—"straight across."

Jackie lifts down a plastic tray; inside is a cross section of a lower leg that looks something like a slice of ham, with two bones, the muscle compartments, the arteries, veins and nerves, as well as the covering of fat and skin—all awash in fluid. I ask her how these were made.

"We froze her, then made the cuts one inch apart. We used a band saw, the kind you use for food."

Four students have seen these exhibits and joined us for a closer look.

"Boy, these are clear," one says. "Why don't we *use* these?"

"We could never get these in a form we wanted. These are just in glycerol [the covering liquid]. We wanted to put them in plastic, so they'd be permanent and easily used, but we couldn't perfect the technique. There are commercial ways to do this, but it's way too expensive for us."

I try to imagine sections in plastic, sort of like Frisbees, or gigantic anatomic poker chips.

Back in the first room, Tassos is cutting by himself at Table 2, while Karen and Konny are at work at Table 5. The other four corpses lie under white plastic, their heads propped up on the wooden blocks. In Karen and Konny's specimen, the eyes were missing, so that all the structures behind the eye lead, in their phrase, "to nothing." Nonetheless they dissect the area for demonstration.

"This is the last dissection for Team A!" Tassos exults, as he trims at the back of the eye. The human eye is larger than we commonly think, since we see only a fraction of it through the lids. The entire eyeball is about the size of a golf ball. Except for a protuberance to the rear, it is very nearly round and covered entirely by the same white sclera we see between the eyelids.

"You know a lot about this, right?" I ask him, recalling that he is finishing a Ph.D. in physiology with a dissertation on the eye.

"Well, the front of the eye, yes, but not the back," he replies. Given the specialization in medical sciences, Tassos knows a hell of a lot about the biochemistry of the fluid in the anterior chamber of the eye and its possible relation to the development of cataracts and glaucoma, but not so much about the structures he is untangling to the rear. He and the two women agree this is a tough dissection, given the crowded complexity of the eye and the fat-embedded nerves behind it.

Dr. Richard Margeson is a lab instructor today, but there isn't much for him to do. He could easily leave early, but I see him pulling a lamp up to the head of a table and turning back the coverings. He sits on a stool, in the same position as the students, and turns his attention, probe in hand, to the head and face of the cadaver before him. Evidently he is giving himself a review of the structures of the head and neck. He has told me that most of his surgery is in the torso and that he tends to remember structures more spatially than by name. He doesn't *need* to do this review, I suspect. But as he makes himself comfortable, I think of someone settling down to a good novel or perhaps a fine meal. Or, to change the image, he is a musician, about to practice his scales.

Unexpectedly, Jonathan appears in the door, but doesn't come in. He seems to be hesitant—not his usual presentation.

"What's happening, ace?"

"Come here a sec. . . . I want you to meet my mother."

I move forward and see Mrs. Kalish, visiting from Chicago. After introductions, Jonathan leaves to find Dr. English for permission to bring her into the lab to see his cadaver. Mrs. Kalish is a lawyer; among her recent cases are some with medical aspects. I wonder how many parents come to visit the cadavers their children have dissected; she's the first I have seen this year.

We make small talk for a moment, but Jonathan is quickly back with permission, and we all enter the lab. Mrs. Kalish puts on a pair of gloves and Jonathan's lab coat over her handsome traveling clothes. Jonathan unveils the cadaver at Table 3. As he talks, he doesn't use the phrase "Little Old Lady"; this term appears to have lost its application. Jonathan pulls back the final coverings, and Mrs. Kalish sees the heavily dissected face. She leans toward it, as if to match her face with the cadaver's.

"Now what can you tell me about her face?" she asks, leaning against the table.

"Well, she's got pretty blue eyes," Jonathan says, squeezing open a pair of lids.

"Why is the eye not clear?" she asks. Tassos, at the next table, can answer this one.

"At death, there's no more ATP to transport chemicals out of the tissues. The cornea swells up and gets cloudy."

"Dear old girl," Mrs. Kalish says. "How did she die?"

"CVA, we are told. Cerebrovascular accident—probably a stroke, although we'll probably never find any direct evidence of that."

"But you've seen evidence of death in other cadavers, yes?"

"Oh sure. There's a cancer patient in the next room no one could miss—the lungs look like they're full of a thousand mosquito bites."

Dr. Marla Luskin, one of today's lab instructors, joins us, and she and Jonathan show parts of the head and skull to Mrs. Kalish.

"And she's a hundred and one years old, you said?" Mrs. Kalish asks. "Bless her heart. She gave her best," she adds softly, as if to the cadaver. Mrs. Kalish pats the blanket and plastic just below the chin, a gesture she has surely made many times tucking in the bedclothes for her own five children, including Jonathan, who now towers over six feet tall beside her.

"Where's your brain, honey?" she asks him.

Jonathan pulls, from beneath the sheets, the six-quart Tupperware container with the brain afloat. He pulls out the brain and describes the basic structures, while she marvels at the notion that this was the brain of a woman with a century of life.

"This is fascinating!" she exclaims. "How do you ever leave this place?"

"Well, when it's midnight, and you've been here for hours, and you still want dinner—it's not hard," Jonathan laughs. "Take a look at this." He shows her the brachial plexus with pride, the armpit he and Steve worked on some weeks back.

"Oh, look, you've got all these colorful flags," she says.

"That represents a lotta work, Mom."

Conversation continues, particularly between Mrs. Kalish and Dr. Luskin, since Jonathan is tidying up some of his work space. The women discuss how the brain works, connections to diet, and implications for some of the clients in Mrs. Kalish's law practice. I admire the ease and practicality of the conversation.

Eventually it is time to leave.

"This was such a treat!" Mrs. Kalish exclaims, as she and Jonathan go out the door.

I watch them leave, thinking about the procession of generations. Jonathan and my daughter are in the younger generation; Mrs. Kalish and I are of the same generation. Are her parents alive, I wonder: that older generation is dying out, sooner (like my father) or later (like my mother who is still alive) but, in any case, ineluctably. Part of the business of looking at dead people, for the students and for me, is accepting our role as children, the offspring of a cohort that is slowly dying away. However distant or soon, our deaths are also guaranteed. Part of becoming a mature daughter or son is coming to terms with death in all of its forms and making peace with our parents before they (or we) die. Perhaps this never happens completely, and survivors always must deal with some unfinished business. When I went to work at my first real teaching job, my father was still on his deathbed. This was a hard but necessary departure for me. Ten weeks later he died, and I came back home for the memorial service. I think I had said sufficient good-byes during the summer that I nursed him, but I never saw his body in the last weeks of his life or after his death. (One of the points of a long wake is the legal need for the community to see that the dead person is in fact dead and that he or she isn't alive elsewhere; another is a psychological demand to know of the person's death *for sure,* to have absolute closure.) Hence my search here in the lab, where I find my lost father in these donated cadavers and come to terms with the journey of his body.

BISECTING THE HEAD

• • •

T HE LECTURE TODAY is on the pharynx and larynx, two odd names
for structures of the throat. Dr. Marla Luskin leads us through some
of the basic but "difficult geometry," in her phrase, that allows us to
breathe, to swallow, and to speak and sing (or "phonate," in medical language). A variety of muscles, some thin, some circular, some very tiny (especially for the vocal apparatus) work together in sophisticated coordination
in this very small area.

About halfway through the hour, she turns the podium over to Dr. Ger-
ald Gussack, an otolaryngologist—a specialist in the ear, pharynx, and larynx. He reviews the structures of the vocal cords and their surrounding
supports, and shows us some striking slides and videotapes of the cords in
action, as seen through fiberoptics. Some of the cords are more gray than
others, the result of smoking. One set of cords is his own; the slide was taken
yesterday. Some film displays—and we hear—a young woman's vocal cords
vibrating while she sings "God Bless America." The two white bands waver
symmetrically under stroboscopic lighting that shows them slower than their
actual 120 vibrations (for some notes) per second. The students applaud
loudly.

"It's really a lot of fun," Dr. Gussack says. "I just basically apply what you
learn here."

One student asks how men's voices change.

"We don't know for sure, but we think there are hormonal receptors

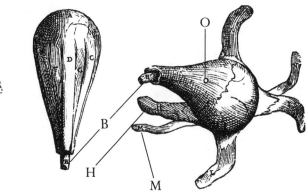

THE EYE: THREE VIEWS

(Figure 27)

From *De fabrica,* pages 238, 239.

THE LEFT-HAND figure shows the right eye in place. The tear glands (hidden behind the top left of the figure) provide moisture for the upper lid to distribute across the eyeball, cleaning and lubricating the surface of the eye. The encircling muscle shown here is the obicularis oculi.

The middle figure shows the removed eye ("looking" upward) with most of the muscles that give it motion in its socket, the fat behind the eye, and the optic nerve ("B"—below). These muscles work in extraordinary coordination, for example in the act of reading.

In the third view, the six muscles that move the eye are dissected free, and readily identifiable as the muscles we know today.

Saunders and O'Malley (page 124) observe a minor error in linking two of the muscles to the left, the superior oblique ("M") and the superior rectus ("H"). They say that the real blunder, however, is the depiction of a seventh, conical muscle ("O") found only in some mammals, such as cattle, but not in humans. Evidently Vesalius failed to follow his own philosophy of using human models exclusively.

in the larynx that are turned on at puberty, causing thickening of the true vocal cords," Dr. Gussack replies.

Upstairs, Team A readies for their last presentation. A student from the next room sits on a stool, with a latex glove stretched over his head; the little stubs of the fingers stick up like a rooster's comb. On the tightly stretched rubber, some of the vessels and nerves of the scalp are brightly rendered in green and red lines. He is hiding in his room so that he can surprise the lab instructor who will hear his presentation in the next room. He sits on a stool and grins, looking wonderfully silly, with his rubber rooster's crest about three inches above the actual, bony crista galli (crest of cock) in his own skull.

The usual routine is underway: Team A practices presentations while the other students listen. Cliff and David are all ready, even with their special treasure, the ethmoid sinus sac still intact. There is one other unusual find, an artificial lens they found in the eye of their cadaver, crystal clear, with two brackets of fine wire to hold it in place. By contrast, the other, natural lenses tend to be cloudy or even tan or yellow, because of cataracts.

"We thought it was the original equipment at first, and said, 'Wow, this lens was in really good shape!'" David says. "But it soon dawned on us that this was an implant, especially when we found the wire clips."

At Table 2, Tassos is preparing to cut an eyeball open. It is somewhat soft. In life, the internal pressure would keep it tauter, hence harder and rounder. The usual white color of the sclera (the white of the eye) extends around the entire globe. The stubs of the six muscle attachments break the round outline, and, to the rear, there is a protuberance of white tail, the optic nerve and its sheath, now trimmed off. Thus the whole assemblage looks like a small white onion, with its stalk cut close. (See Figure 27, above.) The iris (brown in this case) and the dark pupil sit on the front, looking smaller than usual in the context of the entire globe. The pupil is "apparently dark," in the dictionary's phrase, having no actual color. When we see a person's pupil as a dark disk, we are actually seeing into the eye itself, from which no light is reflected back. Still, the structures before me on the stainless steel are recognizably the concentric circles of a human eye now oddly adrift, unmoored from its protective cavern.

Tassos cuts the eyeball open with a scalpel, and the vitreous humor inside spills out, a clear jelly. The retina collapses downward like a tiny rag. The delicacy of these inner structures reminds me of exotic tropical aquatic life in the coral reefs of the skull. "The eye is truly amazing," Tassos says. The cut halves of the eyeball lie on the stainless-steel rail, its liquid spilled. This is a day of endings: it is hard to imagine that the cadavers have much of the human left in them.

Not many of Team B students seem to have read the syllabus description for today's dissection, although they know the job is to "bisect the head," in the phrase from the syllabus that they seem to enjoy repeating. These words have a pleasing solidity, a nice assonance of the repeated "eh" sounds, and a nice rocking rhythm. Like "popping a cadaver," the phrase makes light of the act itself: cutting the skull, vertically, into halves. To "bisect" suggests some neat, geometrical activity, like drawing a line through an angle with a sharp pencil. But in this case, everyone knows the action is, well, ferocious . . . bizarre . . . outré—what *is* the right word? Some of the students hope that they will not personally have to do this.

"Will the instructor come around with that saw again?" I hear several wondering.

Dr. English has mentioned to me that some students in this course, often women, had never sawed anything, ever, and that a skull is not the easiest object to learn to saw upon. Nonetheless, the leader in today's sawing is Dr. Marla Luskin, the lecturer from the past hour, who, in her red dress, high heels, and lab coat, turns out to be a terrific sawyer of skulls. Most of the men are bigger than she is, but she saws first and with a forthright attitude, providing a model. "She's really cool," one student tells me.

She starts at Table 1 and shows them how to angle the open top of the head on the table so that the saw can cut the front of the skull and the back simultaneously. The skull is open at the top, from the previous dissection, like a deep bowl. The cadaver is faceup, although the face is not really much of a face anymore. It is pretty well stripped of skin and fat; by contrast, the ears seem enormous—whorled wings, but appearing as too high on the sides of the cut-down skull. In some cases where the eye has been removed, you can see directly through the orbit—from either direction. Previously, the intact skulls looked like the heads of persons, enclosures for human consciousness. Now there is clearly *nobody there.*

"The cut needs to be just off the midline of the head," Dr. Luskin says, and pulls her saw down slowly, to score the frontal bone, just as any of us in our basement or garage might start the cut on a two-by-four. This illusion is reinforced by her saw, a regular carpenter's cross-cut, with a mottled blade and a wooden handle, whimsically incised, a pattern I remember from the saws in my father's workshop. This saw is not only old, but dull. As a student later puts it: "I could saw just about as well with an umbrella."

Larry and John hold the head as still as possible, while she saws away from the end of the table. Bone dust trickles through the air where the brain used to be, and a crowd of students closes in on this strange scene, including those students who will soon saw other skulls.

"Not something you see every day," says one laconic man.

"That's harsh," says another.

"This is goddamn insane," says another under his breath. "I can't believe it. Sawing the fucking head right in two!"

As the saw cuts down through the forehead in front, and the occiput in back, it also "cuts" through the brain-vacated space in the skull. In all of this strange iconography, the last remnants of humanness of the cadavers are obliterated. A few weeks ago, "reanimation" was a brief theme, but this theme is totally gone now. Larry and John pull the two sides of the head apart, as the thin bones at the base of the skull crack and pull apart. Finally they are down to the first cervical vertebra, which they attack deep in the neck with a scalpel.

"Be careful," Dr. Luskin admonishes them. "I saw a student stab himself once and have to have hand surgery." This comment gets their attention, and they become more careful. Before long, they have enough soft tissue out of the way to turn to a hammer and chisel. A few blows, and the first cervical vertebra comes apart. (This uppermost vertebra, because it holds up the globe of the head, is traditionally called the "atlas" vertebra; the word *verte-*

bra means "something to turn on," indicating the twisting flexibility of the spinal column.) The jawbone is now the only bony structure holding the two cloven parts of the skull together.

At a neighboring table Tim and Saeed saw away, taking turns. The work is taxing, cutting a round, hard surface of a head that they can't keep still. They take a break, leaving the saw stuck halfway through the head, halfway down, to about the level of the nose. Jonathan points at this strange sight, slowly shaking his head. He and Steve mutter about horror movies and Steve Martin's *The Man with Two Brains*.

Charlie, who is from Atlanta, says, "Hell, I could have saved us all a lot of time; there's a sawmill not far from here that'd cut these guys in half— chop chop."

At another table, students saw away, until one says, "Oooops, I guess we're through the hard palate." Shortly he works the saw back up through the head and pulls it out. He stares at the saw.

"Hey, look!" he cries. There is a single tooth—an off-white kernel— caught on the saw.

No one knows what to say.

This is truly one of the strangest dissections. The images, sounds, and even smells of bisecting the head raise in all of us emotions of disgust, horror, and dread. Is this dissection a desecration, with crude tools, crude methods, in order to see the inside of the head? Or are these cuts all part of the anatomical enterprise to see, in this case, into the throat cavity from above? I conclude that bisecting the head is but one more way into the intricacy and wonder of the human body. Part of becoming a physician is finding ways of diminishing horrific material, either to the commonplace, or, at least, to something that can be dealt with. In part, we pay doctors to look at the worst things that can happen within our bodies.

At Steve and Jonathan's table the action is now in full swing. Dr. Luskin is helping, and all three take turns, one sawing, the other two holding the head. It's hard work, and soon both men are sweating. It's almost as if four people (one entirely passive) are in some kind of wrestling match. A small crowd gathers. Jonathan and Dr. Luskin concentrate on holding the head still;

Steve swings his arms, shoulders, and back—up and down. He is pumping hard and sweating freely. The observers lean forward, entranced. In one effort too intense to be controlled, the saw jumps out of the head.

"I just hate it when I slip out of the groove!" Steve bursts out, and everyone breaks into nervous raucous laughter at the wildly inappropriate sexual pun.

"Oh, that's great," Keith says. "If I had a hat, I'd take it off!" Further chuckles.

In this world of the dead, slogans and symbols of vitality are necessary: jokes, songs, baseball caps, off-color mnemonics, radios—whatever it takes. The laughter pays tribute to Steve and Jonathan, our class clowns and champions who help keep us all alive in this cavern of death. Keith's tip of an imaginary hat recognizes their role; it is a particularly droll tribute, given the six cadavers lying around us with the tops of their heads trimmed off at the hat line.

At the next table Tim and Saeed saw steadily downward, and pull the two sides of the head apart. This is the first head entirely split in two, and we all crowd around. It's hard to tell which way is up, and someone asks, "What is that back there—neck muscle?"

"It's the tongue," Tim says.

We refocus, reinform our vision, and make out, in this blob of muscle, the tongue, sawn into two pieces, surprisingly large. The tongue tip is just a flap, as we'd expect, but the back and base of the tongue is a large bulb of intersecting muscles, doming and bulging, like an apple cut in half. It's hard to make out other parts of the head immediately—the whole display seems confusing, visually "noisy." But the table is crowded, so I plan to look more carefully another day.

As I leave, Dr. English, Dr. Wolf, and some students are discussing a widely reported operation, a partial liver transplant, at the University of Chicago, from a mother to a daughter. This is the first operation of its kind and one of much promise. These anatomy professors and students are trying to figure out how the blood supply would work in the posterior lateral portion of the liver taken from the mother. For them anatomy *lives*.

TATTERED CARCASSES

· · ·

HURSDAY . . . AND THE pressure mounts. Students have one more regular week of classes ahead of them before exams, plenty of work to finish, and, of course, a tremendous amount of material to review. "I'm ready to quit now," one student says. Particularly in the lab, there is a kind of cumulative fatigue evident today. "I'll be so glad when this is over," say many students.

The program for the Service of Reflection and Gratitude is coming together. Chaplain Shockley's group meets once again to coordinate music, readings, and the order of the service. The students speak of one of their aims, to show their appreciation for the wonders of the body. "Up in the lab, I keep saying *isn't this amazing,*" one student says. Another replies, "Yeah, I know what you mean. All through embryology, I kept saying, *Wow!*" Karl brings prints of a handsome linocut he has made for the covering of the program, a heart surrounded by some words from a poem by John Stone. Everyone likes it, and they give Karl a round of applause. I remember the day he cut the heart out of his cadaver and offered it to me to hold in my hand.

The lecture today is a lecture/demonstration on the ear, particularly the middle and inner ear. Dr. Rizzolo asks us to sit close to the front and adds that he will not take any questions from persons in the last four rows; some students sitting there move forward. He encourages us to follow along with our skulls: we were asked last time to bring the skull from the bone box, pipe cleaners, and a penlight. The inner ear is a tough area, because it is embedded in bone, virtually impossible to dissect, and hard to study at the gross level. The delicate inner structures are tremendously important, not only for hearing but for balance as well. All physicians need to know about the possibility of dangerous, even lethal infections in these hidden canals.

The lecture, then, becomes a challenge of modeling: without direct access to these structures, how can they be suggested so that the audience gains insight into their shape, size, and position? Rizzolo uses a variety of means, the usual projected slides, of course, but still more important are the drawings he makes on the board with colored chalks, a skull in his hand (with penlight and pipe cleaner), language, and even the living skulls of everyone in the room.

"X marks the spot," he says, drawing on the board two intersecting hallways, the basic canals of the ear as seen from above. One arm is the external canal to the outer ear, the one we are all familiar with. Where it crosses the other, the eardrum lies, and within that crossing are the three tiny bones (malleus, incus, and stapes) that carry sound to the cochlea. These are the smallest bones in the body. Deeper still into the head, we reach the internal canal. Here, the cochlea interprets sounds, and the neighboring semicircular canals interpret position and movement of the head and, therefore, balance. Thus the ear is known as a "dual-function" organ. Since we see only the whorled external part (the pinna), we forget that the inner ear keeps us from getting dizzy and falling down. To stand, to walk, to dance—all such activities depend on the inner ear.

In the process of hearing, air waves are converted to mechanical waves and, finally, to fluid waves, with an amplification of some twentyfold, Dr. Rizzolo explains. We listen to this information with our stereophonic ears, generally unaware of their faithful work.

The other intersecting corridor leads to the mastoid air cells toward the rear of the head, and the auditory tube (formerly known as the Eustachian tube) running forward and down into the nasal cavity. This auditory tube helps balance pressure on the eardrum, as anyone painfully appreciates when the pressure is not balanced, for example, during the descent of an airplane.

Upstairs, Steve and Jonathan have been cutting since noon. The skull of their cadaver is split down the middle, and the whorls and cells of the nose and sinuses are visible on the two halves of the head. Today, however, the difficult chore is to dissect in front of the ear, an area known as the infratemporal fossa (literally, "the ditch below the temporal bone"). This is crowded with fragile structures, and these vary between cadavers.

Right in front of the ear is the zygomatic ("yoking") arch; this bone is cut away with bone cutters. The temporalis muscle above and under this arch (we feel it on the side of the head when we chew) comes next. Two saw cuts take off the top of the jawbone, and the picky fun begins.

"Our cadaver is particularly tough because she has a real small face," Steve says. Neither Steve nor Jonathan calls her Little Old Lady anymore; I ask them about this.

"Nope, she stopped being that for us," Jonathan says.

"But he calls her *something else* now," Steve prods with a grin, but Jonathan won't tell me. I suspect a salty phrase that revitalizes him in the midst of these final and disturbing dissections, and although part of me would like to hear the phrase, another part of me is proud of him for *not* telling me, a measure of his sense of decorum.

They struggle with the end of the jawbone, complaining, "There's just no work space here!" Seeing their dilemma, Dr. Wilson lends them a pair of rongeurs, nippers built like pliers. (See Figure 4, above.)

"Just nibble off bits, but do not twist these, or they can be ruined," he says, demonstrating their biting effect. Under pressure of the rongeur, the bone crystals collapse in little explosions, sometimes sending fragments outward in arcs. Steve and Jonathan, in high spirits, enjoy the efficiency of this new tool, and they use it energetically.

"Chew that jawbone down!" they exclaim, and establish a count.

"One, two, three, *rongeur!*" at which point Jonathan squeezes the handles, and bone shards leap from their cadaver's skull. (In French, *ronger* means "to chew or erode away"; *rongeur* means "rodent," as if the metallic jaws were a rat's snout.) Steve takes his turn, and the energetic count resumes.

"One, two, three, *rongeur!*"

It's a picking-fat, searching, and naming-of-discoveries day, slow and meticulous, especially by contrast with yesterday's head-splitting spectacle. When Dr. Luskin comes through, she is hailed as a skull-sawyer extraordinaire. I ask her where she learned her tricks.

"That was the first time I ever did it," she tells me—to my amazement. I too thought she was drawing on past experience.

Students migrate from table to table, putting together techniques, perceptions, even motivations. At one point there's a kind of group sing of "Schoolhouse Rock" tunes from Saturday morning television; I remember my own daughter's delight at these lyrics, so clever they became implants of grammatical structures into young skulls.

"Oh yeah, and remember this one . . ." the students say. They remember the tunes and words about grammar and the federal government with ease. Once again, good teaching seems to stimulate a variety of senses, the way Dr. Rizzolo did in his lecture earlier today or Dr. Silverman did in his William Harvey lecture.

As the day wears on, however, the students experience intense frustration as they search for tiny arteries, veins, and nerves packed into this complex area. I hear comments up and down the labs:

"Everything is so thin in here, it's just about impossible to dissect."

"This is our last dissection. It's time to be ruthless."

Even: "I've had about enough of this anatomy stuff!"

Jonathan shakes his head, "I've been at this four hours, now; I could have seen *The Deer Hunter* in that time." It is an eerily apt comment, juxtaposing that film's climax (the suicide of Christopher Walken's character, who fires a bullet into his brain) with the sawn-open skulls of these cadavers.

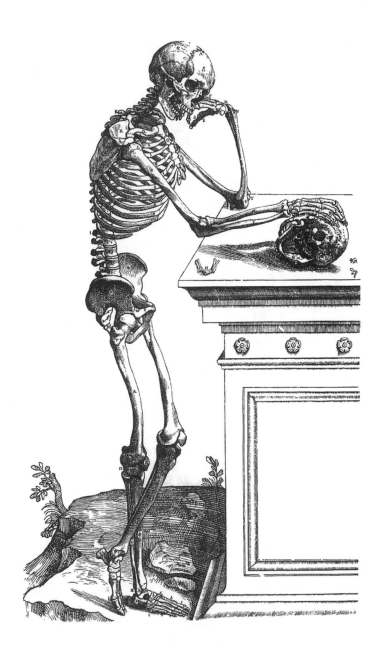

THE SKELETON: SIDE VIEW

(Figure 28)

From *De fabrica*, page 164.

THE SKELETON IS reflectively posed, perhaps considering the *memento mori* of the free skull, although it presumably has no brain to think with. In theme, it is a forerunner of Hamlet and, later, Rodin's *The Thinker*. We might consider the pose a symbolic reanimation of the skeleton.

On the corner of the tomb, the hyoid ("H") bone sits isolated. On the right margin lie two of the ossicles of the inner ear, the malleus (marked *) and, above, the incus (marked with an abbreviation for "que"). Saunders and O'Malley report that some observers felt the images of these bones formed the name of the engraver.

The base of the skull shows the foramen magnum, the large hole where the spinal cord exits the skull to enter the vertebral column.

Vesalius was proud of the illustration, believing that it showed all of the bones of the skeleton simultaneously.

SYMMETRICALLY DESTROYED

. . .

THE LAST WEEK of classes! The students are joyful that the end is near, but depressed at the amount of material—from all three major courses—that they must master before exams next week.

At the final planning session for the Service of Reflection and Gratitude, things go smoothly: the various subcommittees have music lined up, speakers arranged, and texts ready, both for reading and for printing in a booklet. One woman says, "Let me read over the texts so I can desensitize myself. It's okay if I cry here with you, but I don't want to cry in the service."

Another student tells Chaplain Shockley, "Even if the service were never going to happen, I've enjoyed going through this process of planning it."

"We have so much to do, we never have time to think about what it means," another complains.

"Can we meet again in the spring, just for lunch?" someone asks.

Up in the labs, there is much excitement over this last day of dissection. Team B is anxious to present and depart—forever. Team C, with a one-day dissection to do, is eager to get started. It is cold outside today, and winter coats line the hall, draped on top of the embalming tanks.

"I'm so *psyched,*" says Jonathan. "This is the last one!" He is teaching other students at Table 3, going over the structures of the head, split open into two halves.

"Omigod, that's gorgeous!" says one woman, looking at his and Steve's dissection. Jonathan runs a probe up the lacrimal duct from the top of the nasal cavity to the inside of the eye socket. Turning in the volume of the head, his gloved hands are roughly the same tannish gray color of the tissues, as if some animated part of the cadaver were dancing inside the cloven head. When he pulls the two halves of the skull together to show another feature, the bones click together like a large castanet.

It's a cheery day in the labs. The students hum and buzz around the tables, learning from each other, cracking jokes, knowing the end of their labors is near. There are no new threats waiting in the dissections: the throat and ear are considered easy. Furthermore, the cadavers are reduced to fragments. They lie almost entirely encased in white wrappings, with only the remains of the neck and head showing. Faces shredded and skulls split, these remains are hardly recognizable as human. Looking at the six corpses from toe to head, the heads appear to have been cloven by a plow.

As the students stand around the cadavers, their white coats echo the white plastic wrappings on the cadavers; all persons, alive or dead, have the proper uniform.

Kathy and Elizabeth present first and do a good job. "I'll never pick fat out of Nero again!" says Kathy with a smile, going out the door.

Dr. Wilson approaches Table 3, where Jonathan and Steve are ready. Jonathan automatically aims the lights on their exhibit.

Steve begins. "I'd like to present the bony boundaries of the infratemporal fossa," he says, referring to the articulated skeleton hanging nearby. He talks for just under five minutes, including his description of the chewing muscles, the five "muscles of mastication," which move the lower jaw in various ways and push food between the teeth. Steve passes the probe to Jonathan, who picks up the story. They are doing very well. Another five students stand around to hear the result of their dissection.

"I'd like to show you the muscles of the tongue," Jonathan says, and Steve sticks his tongue out and demonstrates the various directions the tongue can move, owing to the three principle muscles that originate in bones and fuse into the tongue (the extrinsic muscles), as well as the three directions of muscle fiber that are in the tongue itself (the intrinsic muscles). Everyone smiles as Steve's tongue shows the moves that allow us to eat, to talk, to kiss, to clean our teeth. The tongue works and plays for us, with very little of our conscious attention; only when it's sore, or when damage to a nerve means it can't function, do we become aware of its importance.

As Steve and Jonathan finish up, Dr. Wilson asks them a half dozen questions. They miss the first one, but answer the rest, and get a good mark for their work. In this test of wits Dr. Wilson's tough questions help them define the limits of their knowledge. During this interchange, the room gets quiet, since the other students want to hear how they do. I feel that the other students, without looking up from their cadavers, are pulling for Jonathan and Steve. One student tells me later that Dr. Wilson's questions are helpful in letting the students know what they still need to master for the exam.

Because other students who didn't do this dissection still want to learn, Jonathan and Steve stick around and demonstrate the structures again. Steve exults, "I am never going to do this again! But actually it was pretty neat!"

"How do we do this?"

"I have no idea."

The members of Team C are taking over, and they find a sorry mess on their hands. Team C did the careful job on the neck a few weeks back, when the head was atop the stalk of the neck. Now things are much changed.

"I can't recognize a damn thing here, and I *did* the neck!" Alex complains, looking at the cadaver. It's the same at all the tables. How do you get oriented to a head that's been plowed in two?

Jocelyne and Lisa take over at Table 3. They have two jobs at hand, to investigate the throat and the inner ear. In order to enter the throat from the rear, they must continue the split of the head, so that it will detach from the spinal column. As some muscles will still hold the halves of the head, this is not technically a *decapitation,* I suppose, but then there isn't much of a head to cut off, either.

"Why is this mandible *here,*" Charlie complains at his table, looking at half a jawbone lying on the shoulder. He has made the required cuts so that the head halves flop forward and to the sides. The neck bones, covered with thin muscles and tissues, have become the end of the cadaver, since the split head is flopped forward onto the chest.

"Looks just like a monster turkey," observes one of the cutters at Nero's table. (While all other cadavers have lost their names, Nero still retains his, owing, I take it, to his singularity and to the particular relationship his students have with him.)

The actual tube of the throat lies bare and pulled forward; the students will dissect the throat from the rear. The tongue lies forward now, split into two symmetrical halves, like a small potato. In corpses where the symmetry is not clear, the students try to match the two halves. One landmark is defined by the horns of the hyoid bone, one of the strangest bones in the human body. Hyoid means "U-shaped," which it is. (See Figure 28, above.) You can feel it—in the front of your neck, about an inch under your jawbone, with its "U" opening to the rear—by probing and pinching with thumb and forefinger on the two sides. If you probe from just one side, the bone will slide away from the touch. Here's why: the hyoid is the least connected of all human bones. It has no joints, no neighboring bones to stabilize it; it hangs by an ingenious system of muscles and is the origin of the hyoglossus muscle, which runs up into the tongue. The hyoid also helps anchor the larynx below. (Once you have the hyoid located, wiggle your tongue from side to side and feel the hyoid's delicate anchoring.)

Students, then, locate the horns of the hyoid (now pointing toward them, as they work at the end of the table), and start to snip into the throat. They cut through the upper constrictor, a circle of fan-shaped muscle that squeezes food downward. That opened, the epiglottis becomes clear, a sturdy flap that looks like a small shoehorn. Its job is to fold down over the trachea (the air tube) so that food from the mouth dumps into the esophagus (the food tube). If this doesn't work, we cough like hell.

At this point, I am tired of looking only, and ask for a glove. Charlie indicates his glove box in a plastic bag. "Grab a feel," he urges. Eagerly, I pull on a glove and trace the inside of the skull and the nasal septum, with its scrolled conchae—these are light and delicate whorls where air we breathe in is warmed and humidified. I feel the tongue (rubbery and tough), the insides of the cheeks, and the horns of the hyoid. I bend the cartilages of the nose and flip the uvula (the word means "grape"), the dangling protuberance at the back of the soft palate. The head is rich with these little, highly specialized structures, and how much they do for us! I end at the epiglottis, bending it down, while my own throat unconsciously swallows, in living parallel.

By looking into the stiffer air tube, the trachea, I can see the vocal folds primly together, the position used for "bearing down" (in childbirth, grunting, moving bowels) and, of course, for speaking.

At the next table, Jim and Margaret work on their cadaver. Jim uses a rongeur to open the bone at the base of the skull, so that he can see the ossicles of the inner ear. He points them out in place, later placing the malleus, which means "hammer," on a wood block. About a quarter of an inch long, it looks like a top-heavy numeral 7. (See Figure 28, above.)

It's a brisk day, and the students chatter and visit. They joke about being finished with anatomy, or even skipping this dissection. One student says, "I don't think we're looking at sixes for this dissection." Another says, "I wanted to calculate whether I could pass if I took a zero on this. I could go home now!" Despite these declarations of freedom, the speakers continue to cut.

TAKE A WALK THROUGH . . .
• • •

I'S FREEZING COLD when I walk to work this December morning, and the lake I pass has a sheet of ice across it. The ice is thin—and will surely soon disappear—but it's the clearest sign of winter I have seen here yet. I throw sticks and rocks out on the ice and watch them skitter across. The larger rocks break through; the smaller ones make a loud, pinging sound, out of proportion to the size of the rock. The ice is a giant eardrum, magnifying sound. I think of Thoreau's Walden Pond, which he imagined to be earth's eye.

Today's lecture is the last regular lecture, a review of the cranial nerves (On Old Olympus Towering Tops . . .). I sit with Cliff and David, who follow along closely, testing wits with the lecturer, Dr. John McDonald. He reviews the nerves, their distributions and function, lacing his account with questions to the students, such as, "And this lower branch supplies the *what?*" Cliff and David—and the others—call out the answers, usually correctly. Several students check details in their atlases. Some students even challenge Mc-Donald on fine points.

Sometimes he responds with such words as, "Technically, you're right. What we're giving you here isn't the whole story, but for the purpose of this course, we will divide innervations as I said." He also says that detailed research in this area could discover a lot more. Thus the students (or some of them, at least) are outgrowing this introductory course and seeing its limits.

McDonald ends with a discussion of cranial nerve IX, the glossopharyngeal and its innervations of the parotid, tongue, and pharynx. He then changes moods, from technical and informative to avuncular and supportive. "Drawing on my own studies, I'll offer you a hint on how to learn some of this material. Pretend that you're taking a walk along the path of a nerve, and just walk yourself through the distributions and their functions. Say, 'I'm walking along from the brain, exiting through this foramen, or that meatus. I then split up with such-and-such branches, or I hitch a ride with this vessel or other nerve. I pick up these components, and reach this or that ganglion before finally branching into these tissues.' " Dr. McDonald says such envisioning of the pathways can help a lot in learning and remembering the anatomy. The students pay close attention; here is a veteran giving the benefit of his own training, offering a proven model.

Back in Dr. Silverman's lecture on the heart, we had the notion of the *Fantastic Voyage,* a movie with a miniature submarine whizzing around in the bloodstream. While this notion was memorably dramatic, I see in Dr. McDonald's model a shift from the dangerous journey to a domestic story, a stroll through a local park's familiar landmarks. As in the learning of other complex activities—driving a car, playing bridge, typing up text—the structures are strange at first, but eventually familiar to the point of automatic functioning.

After the lecture I see Jonathan and Steve, rare attenders of anatomy lectures in the second half of the course, but present today. "We wanted to put in a cameo appearance," Steve says. "I sat in the front row. I even asked a question!"

The next day is the formal review session for the last of the course. Steve and Jonathan attend once again, as, it appears, does the entire class. Dr. English explains the schedule for the four groups to take a walk through the lab exam next Tuesday morning; Dr. McDonald's notion for review will be realized in performance soon enough. By now, the routine is so well known that there are no substantive questions. Dr. English mentions that he has had a "barrage of questions" about the innervations of the pharynx and larynx. Are they branches of the accessory nerve or branches of the vagus nerve? He says that the scientific literature is, in fact, ambiguous on the nature of this division. "More research is needed on this topic; perhaps some of you will do it," he concludes. Today, at least, anatomy is *not* a dead field.

We proceed to our last mock exam, in the same format as before: the tagged exhibit beside the question and five choices. Fifteen pairs of slides take us through the muscles, nerves, blood vessels, and dural folds, the structures emphasized in the last several dissections of the foot, head, and throat. The mood is more informal this time than for either previous review, and students discuss some of the answers with their neighbors as the slides flash by.

"And I understand there are a few more slides to see," Dr. English says, as a slide flashes on, showing the blackboard in one of the laboratories, with the following words printed in colored chalk:

MATINEE

SURFACE

ANATOMY

BUDDIES

A series of slides follows, with various students studying or hamming it up. For example:

IT GETS

LONELY

IN THE LAB

followed by photos of Cliff and Robert planting kisses on the "cheeks" of the articulated skeleton. The students whoop and cheer, and the little show ends in joyous applause.

"I can't take any of the credit—or blame—for those," says Dr. English (although between the lines it is clear that he has cooperated with the students who brought them). Then he goes through the correct answers on the mock exam. Responding to a question about the neck, English says, "It would be back here," folding the hanging screen for the slides out toward the audience and pointing behind the screen (i. e., deeper into the neck). In this whimsical breaking of the frame, English symbolically suggests the arbitrariness of the visual media of the course and even their inadequacy to show the full depth of human structures. The students chuckle at his gesture, which reinforces their growing understanding of the conventional nature of this course. English also uses the phrase "the company line," to indicate the formulas for some of the anatomy that both the instructors and, now, the students know are inadequate, although adequate for the final for this class and, probably, their national board exams. We finish twenty minutes early.

Upstairs—the last time we make this transition—there is a noisy jubilation. I can hear more racket than ever as I come down the hall. It's the last day of lab, with Team C's final presentation and *no new dissections to begin!* The students cluster around the ends of the tables where the dissected heads and throats are uncovered and brightly lit. Margaret is bouncing up and down, demonstrating that her single earring of a skeleton has joints that move and shake. It seems to me this ornament states today's theme of *domestication*—bringing the foreign world of anatomy into the familiar realm of the everyday.

I am fascinated by vocal cords today. A lover of vocal and choral music, I must see these little things; further, I must feel them. Once again Karl and Charlie are accommodating and give me a latex glove. They open up the airway of their cadaver and show me the tiny folds, about three-quarters of an inch long (the width of a thumbnail).

"Here's the false cords," Karl says, indicating a thicker, heavier fold above, "and here's the true vocal cords." They are two little strings, edges of the throat that come together to form the two sides, the anatomic basis for flesh to make words. When I think of the sound of a tenor like Placido Domingo or a soprano like Jessye Norman, I find it hard to imagine these tiny, thready folds. With the throat cut apart from the back, the two halves are separated now, forever. What did this man say over the course of his life? To whom did he sing?

I touch one cord: it is highly pliable and readily bends away from my touch. With its supportive structures destroyed, it is inordinately delicate now. In life, it would be stretched to yield vibrations, like a violin string. With two cords working together, to change the musical analogue, it would be a double reed, as in a bassoon. I visit a few other vocal cords, finding them much the same. Even Nero's set, to our amazement, is delicate and small.

At Table 6, I ask Jim whether the cadaver is decapitated. The vertebral column is cut, but the flesh holds together; besides, is this really a head anymore?

Jim blows my caviling right away. "It sure *felt* like a decapitation to do it." His definition brings home the emotional truth of this activity. If we follow Jim's insight, all the Team Cs have done decapitations, committed this strange action under the guidance and protection of medical training. More than one student has said to me, "You know, we could get sent to jail for the stuff we do up here, if we weren't med students." I don't know whether this claim is technically true in any legal sense, but it is valid from a personal and moral standpoint: society allows medical students (and physicians) to break certain taboos that no one else can.

Don Shockley and I fall into conversation at the side of the room on these topics of taboo, criminality, and special permission. His understanding— which he was sharing with students earlier—is that medicine is a *profession* with a particular calling. In the training for this profession, there is a crossing of a line, an initiation into a world with special rights and privileges, as well as duties.

At Table 1, Chris and Dave are getting ready for their presentation. Chris wears a red shirt and a green sweater under his lab coat; Dave wears a T-shirt with red and green splotches. They both wear Santa Claus caps, pointed and red, with white trim. The red is eerie, purplish under the lab's harsh fluorescent lighting. In a room painted mustardy yellow, with a tan floor, and full of white coats and cadaveric wrappings, these hats provide two brilliant points of energy. Chris and Dave pace about, muttering their presentations over and over.

Konny and Karen arrive at Table 5 and cry, in unison, "Where's her head!" They did the neck two weeks ago and see now the final transformation of this cadaver into dissected remains.

Larry plans a keg party on Thursday following all exams, and Jonathan and Cliff go to the window to check on the weather: the Sympathetic Chain Gang is in the semifinals of the football league and will play at four o'clock. I see these topics as part of Real Life, now blending with the anatomy lab. I can't remember anyone standing at the window to discuss the weather before.

At Table 4, Eugene, Mei, Jonathan, and Charlie are telling the story of various nerves and arteries: "It originates here, then dives deep, then courses tortuously . . ." using the standard phrase of the instructors, but making the account, in space and time, their own. It is a version of Dr. McDonald's "Take a walk . . ." and it seems to be working.

Dr. Luskin is ready to hear Chris and Dave in their silly hats. Everyone knows something special is coming, so they crowd around the table and *shush* the room into silence. One student places a portable tape recorder directly on the plastic-covered chest of the cadaver.

"Listen my children and you shall hear / A midnight tale of larynx, pharynx, and ear," Dave resoundingly begins.

"The constrictors were all hung by their origins with care," we learn, and "the palatine tonsils were all snuggled in their beds." Aha! It's an anatomical "The Night Before Christmas." As Chris and Dave roll on through the rhymes and, of course, the anatomical objectives (poking with their pointers in the cadaver), their audience grows, until two dozen students are clustered around, nodding and grinning. The presenters conclude:

> "With your acoustic nerve, you will hear us recite
> 'Merry Christmas to all and to all a Good Night!' "

And the room rings with applause and laughter.

Here is another kind of domestication: the Christmas hats, the poetry, and the season's festivity have reached into this strange room and claimed even the battered head of this corpse as part of the celebration. The anatomy room is no longer some strange room "up there," but a part of these students' lives, and their good energy has, in a sense, taken over the room and embraced all cutting, all anatomy, and all the cadavers into the larger world of the outside. In their delight and validation through applause, the students acknowledge the imagination and goodwill of these presenters' performance and the anatomy made clear. The students now constitute a comfortable society of anatomic adepts.

Almost immediately, another show cranks up, and many of us hurry to the next room to hear Lisa and Gail. Gail wears a man's jacket and a tie under her lab coat: she is a TV host. Lisa has a name tag with LISA on her lab coat, and a carefully drawn and colored sign lies on the cadaver's stomach, JEOP-ARDY: we are to be treated to a variation of the quiz show. Many who heard the Christmas presentation are here now, including Chris and Dave, still in their red caps. They stand at opposite ends of this next table, visual poles of festive energy.

Dr. Wilson verifies their names, and we are ready to go. Kyra holds up the JEOPARDY sign and hums her version of the show's theme song. "Welcome to 'Anatomy Jeopardy,' " Gail proclaims in the exaggerated inflections somehow necessary for television, "and our reigning champion is Li-sa, from At-lanta, Georgiaaaa! What are your hobbies, Lisa?"

"Anatomical dissection and checking formaldehyde levels in the lab!" she enthuses.

"That's great, Lisa, and what category would you like to start with?"

"I'll take the Middle Ear—for an A in anatomy!" Lisa shrieks.

Gail then describes the intersection of the auditory tubes to which Lisa cries out, "What is the tympanic cavity?" according to the idiosyncratic style of the quiz show, where information is identified by formulation of a question.

"Very good, Lisa, and which category is next?"

"I'll go for the constrictor muscles of the pharynx for a year's supply of charcoal masks!" Lisa exclaims.

They work their way through the presentation objectives, with further comic references to the course in the putative awards, including a summer research assistantship with Dr. Wilson, who is listening and assessing their work right now.

"And our *home* television audience can see these *ossicles* of the inner ear," Gail proclaims at one point. The twenty of us watching are spellbound at the wit, the energy, and the quick pace of this presentation. I see grins around the table, as the technical information of anatomy is expertly conveyed by the television idiom—yet another domestication of this foreign world.

"And this is the *last show* of 'Anatomy Jeopardy,' which is being *canceled* due to *poor ra-tings!*" Gail concludes, and the listeners break into whoops and cheers.

Back in Room 1, Lisa and Jocelyne are giving their presentation to Dr. Luskin. They are among the last to present, and the room is emptying out. Although they have been done for a long time, Dave and Chris are still around to teach anyone who wishes to hear about their exhibit. Lisa and Jocelyne finish up, and cover up their cadaver. They leave the light on, which shines brightly on the white plastic over the face. I congratulate them on finishing and they, like the teams on either side of them, depart. The three tables on the window side of the room are now empty of students. The cadavers look much like they did on the first day of the course, long mounds covered by white plastic. Soon, two more tables are finished, their dissectors also gone.

One, Table 6, is still going strong, however, with all six team members reviewing various areas of the body. They have adopted the quiz-show language for rotating the leadership of the review ("our next contestant"—applause). They're having a great time, much like a group of old friends around a poker table or a game of Monopoly. Except for them, the room is empty. Five cadavers lie under their neat white coverings, as they did sixteen weeks ago.

. . .

One light is still on, at Table 3, where I did most of my observation. The cadaver, its job finished, lies under the plastic. It (not she) will serve one more function, the anatomy practical exam, but the daily work of dissection is complete. I turn off the light at Table 3 and leave.

WE DON'T STACK THEM
. . .

DR. ENGLISH HAS invited me to watch the setup of the anatomy lab practical exam, so I show up at Monday noon, as he and Dr. John McDonald start to lay out the typed questions on an embalming tank in the hall. They have twenty-five questions and a few spares. Their job is yet another version of an anatomical treasure hunt: to find good exhibits for the exam. It takes them about two hours, often because they further dissect (or even dissect from scratch) an area they want to be clear or "classic," as they say, in its presentation. It is a pleasure to watch them work: they are nimble in their trimming and labeling, clearly at a higher level of skills than students. "Well, at least *it doesn't look like a dog's dinner,* as my colleague used to say," Art acknowledges.

I talk with John, who is working on a cervical nerve. I mention the 101-year-old cadaver at Table 3. "Is that how long you plan to live?" he asks me.

"Not real likely. The men in my family tend to die early," I say. "How about you?"

"Not a chance, with all the pollutants in the world, not to mention the ones I work with every day in the lab."

I wonder to what extent such notions have any influence on our eventual health and death. Just in case, I resolve to live a long time, in optimal health.

Art tags a muscle on one cadaver, a nerve on another, then a blood vessel. With twenty-five stations to set up, the two men keep hustling. "They'll hate this one," Art says cheerfully, labeling a part of an infratemporal fossa.

We hear noises in the hall and look up to see six or eight people all dressed up, with strange looks on their faces as they peer into the labs. One person talks animatedly, waving his hands toward the cadavers.

"These damn tours," Art mutters. "I keep asking the third-years *not* to bring prospective students by here. We are *not* a freak show!" he says, with passion.

"Why do they persist?" I ask.

"I imagine because anatomy was such a rite of passage to them. These labs show the major separation between them as third-years and any pre-meds."

The next morning is the lab practical. The weather is nasty, cold, and rainy, with a forecast of sleet and maybe snow by evening. I see students headed for the anatomy building carrying black suitcases. They look like band students, except that they'd all be playing only two instruments: the large cases hold half a skeleton; the small ones (more like lunch boxes) hold a single skull. Today is the last day to return these valuable items.

Upstairs, the lab instructors are arranging answer sheets, pencils, rest stations, and the like. The first batch of twenty-eight students is assembling by the elevator. They make a quite a hubbub—no shy beginners here. They are the first of four groups today. Dr. Luskin has put out a box of chocolates with a note wishing these M-1s good luck. Jim Wilson meets each group and goes over the rules. He usually says, "As before . . . ," since this is the third exam, and the students know the routine. As each group heads down the hall, I hold up a sign, MORAL SUPPORT, to which they respond with laughter, high fives, and the like.

"No *im*moral support?" asks Steve as he goes by, grabbing my hand.

Jon Stahlman calls out, "We brought home the championship!" It takes me a moment, but I grasp that he means the intramural football championship. I like his use of the word *home.*

The students are wearing jeans, sweat clothes, running shoes, and duck boots. There is an assortment of hats and scarves, today: Dave wears his Santa's hat with two buttons (KEEP SMILING and LEAVE ME ALONE——I'M HAVING A CRISIS); Mike wears a smooth Panama hat; Jocelyne has on a beret; Steve has a strange leather cap of unknown origin and purpose; Jonathan wears his perennial, dirty white baseball cap with the brim pointing upward at a forty-five-degree angle. There are a dozen or more caps throughout the morning, many of them worn backward or flipped up. Several men are growing beards. While the students all have on their required lab coats, their personalized dress underneath claims their independence. Lisa Drake has a Christmas sweatshirt under her coat. Margaret is wearing her skeleton earring on one ear and a large tiger on the other. She explains: "This shows I'm an 'anatomy animal.' "

I watch all four groups, out of loyalty, out of a wish to witness the entire ritual. The students move from station to station with the regularity of the seventy-five-second alarms from the hall, with the regularity of Human Anatomy veterans who have almost completed the course.

On Thursday, their "joint" exam will finish the anatomy course entirely; that afternoon, they have a take-home for community health. Some students are planning on leaving Friday. The new paths open up and out.

As for the cadavers, their path will go like this: in the next two days, their remains go to the basement for temporary storage on trays. Then, in sets of two, they travel to the crematory a few miles away. I learn this from Jim Cooper, the embalmer, who will work on these final dispositions. Jim says the crematorium can't handle more than a few bodies at a time, since the bodies are burned individually to keep the ashes separate. (It takes two or three hours to burn a body and cool the ashes.)

"Besides, we don't stack them," he says. "That's not right."

Even in their final state—cut into unrecognizable forms, with organs removed and heads sawn in half—these cadavers are treated with respect and as the remains of the individual donors. Thinking of my father's body and perhaps my own (should I choose to give my body to a medical school), Jim's promise of care is deeply comforting.

REFLECTION AND GRATITUDE
• • •

I'S COLD AND dark, windy and wet, but about seventy-five students and all of the faculty are at the chapel at 7:00 P.M. for the Service of Reflection and Gratitude. Many have dressed up in suits or dresses, but some have come directly from the med library, where, dressed in jeans and sweatshirts, they have been studying for their other exams. Some are still discussing questions from the lab practical this morning: was that a styloglossus or a glossopharyngeal muscle?

"Through them we touch the body of the world," read the words of physician-poet John Stone on the cover of the program. They are set in Karl Jacob's linocut depicting the heart he removed from his cadaver. (See Figure 29.)

This service is the tenth annual service that Don Shockley and successive classes have put together. "Each one is different," he has told me, "depending on the talents and interests of the classes." Each class has a mixture of belief traditions—Protestant, Catholic, Jewish, Buddhist, agnostic, secular humanist—but the participants, regardless of background, seem to accept the general notion of "a larger context," and, certainly, the notions of reflection and gratitude.

The interior of Cannon Chapel is decorated with greenery and red bows for the Christmas season. Although the building itself is large, the worship space is relatively small, with seating on three sides of a central area.

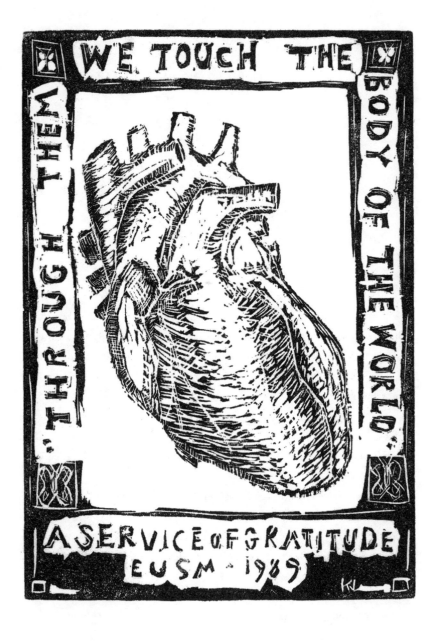

"Through Them"

(Figure 29)

THIS LINOCUT, BY first-year medical student Karl Jacobs (used by permission) was the cover for the program of the 1989 Service of Reflection and Gratitude. The text is from an unpublished poem by John Stone written for an earlier service.

The heart displays the great vessels that must be severed in order to remove it from the body.

Thus the space seems comfortable, more homey than institutional. On the other hand, this is an official part of the university, and there is a symbolic sponsorship, especially through the work of the chaplain, who, in a sense, is ministering to all of us through this service.

Dave, Paul, and Rogena walk to the front with their trombones and play a trio while we take our seats. Linda follows with a flute solo. Don Shockley takes the podium to greet us and to remind us of the purposes of the service. We all know these, of course, but his reminder is a part of the ritual: his words about reflection and gratitude finally make real this long-awaited service, this formal and celebratory end of the Human Anatomy lab. He also asks us to hold any applause until the end. In this three-quarter round setting, the mood is informal: we can see each other and we are *not* wearing lab coats.

Wade walks to the podium and slowly reads from Psalm 139:

> For thou didst form my inward parts,
>   thou didst knit me together in my mother's womb.
> I praise thee, for thou art fearful and wonderful. . . .
> Thou knowest me right well;
>   my frame was not hidden from thee,
> when I was being made in secret,
>   intricately wrought in the depths of the earth.
>   —Ps. 139: 13–15 (R.S.V.)

Suddenly this text has new meanings, as I think of the musculature, the organs, the connections of nerve and artery we have seen. I feel twinges in my eyes and nose—the intricate lacrimal apparatus I have recently seen—now making tears.

Next at the lectern, Gail and Shelena take turns reading from Leonardo da Vinci's *Quaderni d'Anatomia,* the section called "The Order of the Book":

> This depicting of mine of the human body will be as clear to you as if you had the natural man before you. . . . But you must understand that this amount of knowledge will not continue to satisfy you, seeing the

very great confusion that must result from the combination of tissues with veins, arteries, nerves, sinews, muscles, bones, and blood, which of itself tinges every part the same colour. . . . In the same way there will be put before you three or four *demonstrations* of each limb. . . .

Thus, in *fifteen* entire figures, you will have set before you microcosm. . . .

— *The Literary Works of Leonardo da Vinci,* ed. Jean Paul Richter, 3rd ed., vol. II (London: Phaidon, 1970), pp. 87–88, emphasis added

As they read, the women emphasize "demonstrations," which reminds us of the presentations, and "fifteen," the exact number of the dissections. I hear chuckles in the audience.

Then a series of students read their own tributes and memories. They don't walk up in front but rise at their chairs in the audience and stand amidst their peers. Since they are scattered through the crowd, their voices suggest an expression of ideas and feelings of the entire class.

Terry reads her poem, "To a Medical Student," in which the cadaver speaks to her, giving bones, ligaments, and sinews as a "final offering" to help sustain further life.

Bill Paxton invokes the "generosity, courage, and foresight" of the persons who gave their bodies for medical education.

Grace thinks about the semester with her cadaver, Lillie, and concludes that "The very fact that she bequeathed her human form indicates that her choices in life were for the enrichment of others."

Raju describes a dream he had of a walk with his cadaver; he felt that "she understood my immense respect for her."

Renae sees both the "anonymous gift" and the life her cadaver must have had: "Thin muscles and frail bones belie the person who once slept, ate, laughed, loved, and cried as we."

Lisa Drake finds "the laying on of hands / Has taught me more than entire rooms / Of professors ever can."

And Steve remembers the camaraderie of the twelve "A-teamers" in the room he worked in. For him, the empathy extended laterally, so to speak, among his colleagues.

These students read well, and their classmates turn their heads to hear each in turn. I see nods of assent and hear muttered *yeses*. I remember the remark of one student: "They make us work so much we don't really have time to think about what it all means." Finally we have time and space to reflect and evaluate.

Joan plays a movement from a Vivaldi flute concerto, accompanied by Mimi.

Dr. Marla Luskin presents the first of two faculty perspectives. She says that although she was one of the instructors for the course, she feels that the real teachers were the cadavers themselves. She goes on to describe two emotional countermovements: first, a depersonalizing of the cadavers during the course, so that work was possible, but, second, a placing of the cadavers back into contexts of life and death.

Now it is my turn. I have listened and watched a long time; the students have asked me to report on what I have seen and heard, even though I am not regular faculty. I am nervous about the job, but I am glad to step behind the podium and open my folder. I look around the large U of audience and start to read:

TRIBUTE TO THE HUMAN ANATOMY CLASS

I have been your guest for the past sixteen weeks, listening to the lectures and looking over your shoulders in the laboratory. You have been kind and open to me about your work, and I thank you for these courtesies. It is now my job to try to assemble words that will adequately give witness to the journey you have taken; these brief remarks are a start.

It is an unusual privilege to look into the marvels of the human body, an opportunity very few people ever have. I remember the words and phrases you used—*awesome, wonderful, that's so cool, what a miracle*—as you worked your way through the abdomen, the pelvis, the brachial plexus, and the head itself.

But there have been many moods on this trip, from disgust and repugnance to elation and wonder, from jokes and high spirits to fatigue and depression. I can think of few parallels in postgraduate studies that take you, as individuals and as a class, through such a rich and difficult experience. It's a major step in your formation as doctors: becoming able, on the one hand, to confront the difficulty—even the horror—of a disintegrating body; learning, on the other hand, to work—with pleasure—with the complex majesty of the human body.

In a sense, you have been journeying through a valley of death, confronting questions of human limits and mortality. Each cadaver is a mirror: of our grandparents, of our parents, and of ourselves. Whether our own bodies ever go to anatomy labs or not, they surely will disintegrate, one way or another. In a society that is neurotically afraid of death, to deal—firsthand—with a corpse is a crash education in death: *you have seen and considered some of the absolute limits of humanity.*

As you emerge from this strange, difficult, even wonderful experience, I see you as richer and fuller persons, more willing to understand both life and death, more motivated to build your studies around the structures of the body, more prepared to help your future patients.

And so emerges a fine paradox, that out of the cutting and the sawing something beautiful has been built, from the bits of fat, the bone sawdust, the arteries that dried out and broke when you least wanted, from the tatters, the scraps, the ashes of the human phoenixes—the nineteen cadavers that were given to you for your work—a harvest emerges of two things. First, there is, of course, the knowledge that will help you to maintain the health of living bodies. But perhaps equally important are the new resources that will help you in healing yourselves, since you have, in a sense, looked into the abyss, plumbed it, and continued with life; thus there is a new wholeness for you that embraces even death, and this is a step on the path toward wisdom. In this unlikely paradox, of life arising from death, the journey continues.

Walking back to my seat, I hear my heels on the parquet floor. The room is still.

Larry sings "Somewhere" from *West Side Story,* accompanied by Chris Nevins on the guitar. In Bernstein's modern version of *Romeo and Juliet* the song is a kind of elegy; like many songs about death and loss, the lyrics suggest an order, a proper time and place for those who die.

Karl moves to the podium and says he'd like to make a presentation to the Anatomy Department; would Dr. English please come forward? He takes a framed copy of his linocut and hands it to Dr. English, while mentioning the source of the quote and the symbolism of the butterflies in the corners of the print: transformations of living beings, even in death. English holds the frame carefully in both hands as he returns to his seat.

To conclude, Maggie asks us to stand and say the following lines by physician-poet John Stone:

> *Together we are grateful, for we know*
> *the privilege it is to touch another,*
> *whether in the name of science or love.*
> *The touching here has been made up of both.*
> *By their extraordinary gifts*
> *these dead have taught the living how to touch.*

We stand in place, while the three trombonists play a lively gavotte to close the service, and everyone, still standing, suddenly breaks into applause. It is a strong, even, and prolonged clapping, a corporate affirmation of the words, sounds, and images of the service that have represented the complex memories and emotions of the long semester.

In this ritual we have extended—or even added—one more dimension to "the gaze," a spiritual, philosophical, emotional dimension. The strange image of the "spiked slide" comes to my mind, in which Cliff and Bob kiss the skull of the articulated skeleton: while that was primarily humorous, the gesture symbolizes love and care for the dead. I also think of the standing musclemen of Vesalius's text, as if still human and erect in the natural world. By recognizing the spiritual importance of the cadavers, perhaps we erect them once again, reassemble them, resurrect them from their cadaveric fall.

CADAVERS IN SEASON

• • •

(THIRD ESSAY)

WINTER IS SOMEWHAT early this year. The chill is sporadic, as temperatures zoom up and down, but we've had snow flurries twice—well ahead of normal. The Atlanta newspaper trumpets on page one the threats of snow and ice: this southern city has little snow removal equipment, the roads are treacherously built in sinuous twists over the hills, and many of the drivers don't know how to drive on snow. Having lived in Minnesota, I have seen life continue routinely through heavy snows, temperatures below zero, even blizzards. I am tempted to laugh at Atlanta's panic, but in truth I think the southern approach is better: most Americans work too hard, never taking time to think about the meanings and values inherent (or missing) in their lives. If a light snow in an ill-equipped city forces us to stay at home once in a while so that we can ponder our lives, so much the better. Especially in the so-called professions, the practitioners work so obsessively that they have no time to reflect upon what they profess. What faith, what assumptions, what responsibilities, what values and deeper meanings do they see in their work? As several students have said to me, "We spend so much time studying and cutting, we don't have time to think about what it means." This will be, for them, a lifelong dilemma in medicine, and I hope they will find time and space for reflection. Karl said at the reception following the Service of Reflection and Gratitude, "I wanted to take a camera through the anatomy course, just to chronicle all we saw and did, but I never even got it into the lab." His words went off like flashbulbs in my head, analogues to what I wish for my words.

Today, there is another snow, just half an inch, I suppose, but enough to close the schools in four counties. I am at home myself, looking out the window at the gentle white flakes sifting down, and thinking about the ice on the pond nearby. This pond is good-sized, at least a dozen acres, with much of it in the shadow of an imposing hill. Since it is shallow, little warmed by the sun, and protected from rippling winds, it freezes over readily when the temperature falls into the twenties. The sheets of ice build out from the shore, joining in complex crystalline patterns. The new ice branches out into great swirls of fine tracery, like frost crystals writ large.

The last lake I lived with for a winter was in Minnesota, where the ice formed, and formed, and formed, until it was twelve to fifteen inches thick, sufficient for walking across, skating, bonfires, even driving cars. Some northwoods people would push a wrecked car out on the ice and take bets on the date of its final plunge, marking the spring thaw. In Atlanta, the rhythms of freezing and melting are quicker and less dramatic, but, in principle, the same, and these rhythms offer symbolic meaning as I look back over this season in the anatomy lab.

Even before the semester began, the cadavers, through the chemical preservation of embalming, were held back from melting into the world. In their stopover at the anatomy labs, they would take a detour from their natural return to the earth. They are not, however, suspended in ice, visible but imprisoned out of reach forever. Instead, they are actively engaged texts and teachers to the students who cut them, who study them. We use the phrase "suspended animation" to refer to persons in a coma; for the cadavers, it's more like a "suspended disanimation," a stopover between death and final disposition.

The cutting is a step toward the final disintegration of the bodies, a part-by-part disassembling. While some parts leave the immediate wholeness of their body, they (with a few exceptions, mostly minor) are carefully saved for cremation later. With cremation—very likely occurring for some cadavers as I write today—a thawing of sorts dramatically occurs, a rapid oxidation of the parts that will burn, freeing much of the body to the currents and eddies of the sky, from which these gases will join other chemical recombinations of nature: re-embraced, reincorporated. The slow time of the anatomy lab is finally over, and natural cycles resume with a roar of the gas flame. The cremated dead rejoin nature much more quickly than the routinely buried dead, locked in wooden boxes, then sealed in concrete vaults below—but not really in—the earth. I'm happy that my father's remains took the more direct path.

The ashes of the cremated cadavers—bone fragments, chunks, flakes, meal, or dust—will be buried with a service by the medical school, unless they are claimed by families. Some families will bury them in a cemetery plot, while others will scatter them according to some ritual—over a meadow, a stream—likely at a place much loved by the deceased. Even when the ashes are buried in an urn, this "freezing" is not absolute: after a long delay, these elements too will rejoin the enormous cycles of nature.

Our society's attitudes toward death are another kind of ice within the minds of the students, an ice that melts as the students learn. As they become more familiar, more comfortable with a cadaver, they can create their own understandings of the various ends of life and human mortality in general. As their sense of mortality deepens, they also have a richer sense of human vitality and, as well, a richer concept of themselves as future healers who can approach and intrude upon a living human body. The cadaver, although dead, may be the first body that they can—indeed must—medically touch. They are almost surprised that they can do this, without fear of reprisal for committing the crime known as battery. In the anatomy lab, however, they can touch with impunity and they can make the first cut—and then many more. They can—indeed must—invade the body of a fellow human, concretely, specifically, and willfully. Several physicians have mentioned to me this important pivot in medical training as an advancement in both technical skills and in personal feelings about death, touching, and the wonderfully complex activities of the human body.

To work on a cadaver is a step toward working with a living person, when doctors "invade" through touch, through conversation, even in the tender sharing of weakness and pain with patients. The med students have to create their own stability in wisdom to deal with the sickness and debility of their patients. (They'll need to become comfortable working with patients who will be older than they are as beginning physicians, patients the ages of father or mother, grandparent or favorite aunt; social barriers also will need to thaw for these young docs to do their best work.) When the patient says, "It hurts right here, Doc," he or she may mean, "God, it hurts, and I am so frightened. Can you help me? Now?" And the dialogue continues, perhaps to include life-and-death choices. Medical training puts one necessary building block upon another to bring students to professional maturity. The anatomy course is one of the most massive blocks and one of the first: a foundation.

I have seen students stroke the shoulder or forearm of the cadaver as if to say *Thank you for sojourning with me a while; I give you my blessing as you continue on your way.* There is also the explicit good-bye at the end of the course, in the Service of Reflection and Gratitude, where students repeatedly recognized the gifts of bodies to support their learning. By whatever means, the partnership is dissolved, and cadaver and student continue on their appropriate paths. The word *cadaver* indicates, of course, a dead person. If we look at the origin of the word, we find that it means someone who has "fallen" (compare "cadence" in music, a "falling" of chords to rest, to a harmonic home). After falling, the corpse would, in some state of nature, be immediately subject to the external elements (vultures, for example) as well as internal bacteria. One definition of the emergence of humanity in prehistoric times includes evidence of funeral practices, suggesting a sense of cultural responsibility for the dead body within both natural and supernatural orders. To care for a fallen fellow human so that she or he properly enters the next realm is, an anthropologist might say, a civilized act. I think of Antigone's duty to bury her brother. After the downwardness in death, the move to the afterlife, in many cultures, is often upward, to the heavens. And what moves? A soul, a spirit, a vital *pneuma*—cultures differ in concepts, but often we accept a living force beyond the materials of the body. Maybe there is, in fact, only oblivion at death, but isn't it more interesting to consider more? What if our time on earth is as the Venerable Bede saw it, only the brief flight of a bird through a banqueting hall, with longer trajectories before and after?

Even as we assume a soul and hope for such a future, we can do little with concepts or words for the disintegrating remains of the dead. We have an inelegant word in English, *carcass,* generally indicating the slaughtered body of a human or animal, but also, by extension, the tattered wreck of anything—a city, an empire. By the end of the course, the body has become more carcass than cadaver, although neither word seems adequate. When the body has gone past the wholeness we associate with living bodies, we have no vocabulary to explore and assess the wreckage, probably because of the aversions of our culture in the past. Is this because we are unfamiliar with such dissolution, or because our denial of it doesn't allow us to acknowledge it as the inevitable goal of our own bodies? Our estrangement is almost complete. I remember a story told about a mountain rescuer who had to recover the body of a climber who fell to his death on a cliff. The body lay on a narrow ledge, so narrow there was nowhere for the climber to put his feet after rappelling down. As a result the rescuer stepped directly on the chest of the dead man, causing gases of decomposition to exit through the throat and vocal cords, which made a terrible noise and nearly scared the rescuer out of his wits and off of the ledge. The story was told with some gusto, as news of an unknown world, as a gothic vignette to cause a certain shiver among listeners, as an act of tribute for the varieties of experience death may provide. A recent book by Sherwin B. Nuland, *How We Die,* has sold well, probably because it tells of taboo topics we find at once repellent and fascinating, because it offers a vocabulary for what most frightens us.

As the course progresses, the students become aware of their unusual and privileged role to poke and peer among the bodies of the dead. They also begin to wrestle with a dual vision they must develop: first, the disciplined, scientific eye that will help them with their diagnoses and prescriptions, and, second, the intuitive eye of compassion that will help them heal the souls of their patients, even the ones they cannot medically heal. Before the twentieth century, the latter gift was probably the main resource of the physician, along with a small collection of effective drugs, and many of these, such as opium and its derivatives, were merely palliative. As modern pharmacology, surgery, imaging, and many other fields have developed in the last century or so, the emphasis has shifted more to the technical view, and the challenge for wise physicians, for medical humanists, and for society at large is to promote the second kind of vision, the vision of an art of health care that is not only technically excellent but also informed by wisdom of what it means to be human.

What did the students think about the course? I have asked many and received a range of answers. Three are typical. "I loved this; I'm going to be a surgeon." Some students were immediate converts to anatomical enterprise and are ready to build their lives around it, but these are small in number. More common is the second response: "I learned much more than I thought possible," they said, with a variety of emotions. Many felt this way; the human body is now known to them as an intricate marvel, however long or tedious the course seemed. Third is this: "I never did like anatomy that much, but I love the human body." Some students never grew accustomed to the smell, the sight of the dead bodies falling to bits, or the hours of difficult handiwork, but they liked what they uncovered as they went, the discoveries that came through the effort, and the growing understanding of the human body, which will be, in a sense, their working partner for all their professional lives.

The concrete, physical stimuli were unavoidable: the first look into the guts, the sound of the sawing of bones, the smell of the formaldehyde, the spongy feel of lungs. These perceptual impacts were so strong that the students were forced to make interpretations of them. I heard students later saying things like: "Opening the head was so *weird!* I kept seeing it happening again!" And, implied, "What did that mean?"

Two words help bring this all together. The first, *laboratory,* is obvious and needs little comment: the place where labor is done in a concentrated, extended, and disciplined way. The students are hard workers, and they have practiced the work habits that will make them dependable physicians. Equally important, they have learned attitudes of dealing with difficulties. Some of these are technical or mechanical problems, such as cutting out tiny bones of the inner ear. Other difficulties are perceptual and emotional: how to deal with a repugnant cadaver (or an unattractive or hostile patient); how to deal with personal, internal conflicts common to all med students: overload, fatigue, uncertainty, and mystery. As the students have faced these various trials, they learn (or begin to learn) that they have resources to meet such difficulties and that they can support each other.

The other word to bring order from shreds is *season*. This word derives from Latin *satio* or "sowing time," which relates to our modern words *seed* and *semen*. In agricultural societies of the Northern Hemisphere, spring was the time to sow the seeds, summer the time to tend crops, fall the time for harvest, and winter the time for reflection, crafts, and study. The school year in America still typically follows this pattern, even though most students will not work in the fields, come summer. Indeed, industrial societies have largely forgotten the cycle of the seasons that brings food to the grocery store. Considering the agricultural meanings of seasons can help us order the year sequentially and symbolically and can show the procession of life and death. The cadavers, "frozen" in a kind of chemical winter, will be released to rejoin the cycles of the seasons.

If we cut lumber from green trees, we stack it so that it will dry without warping—in order to season it, we say. We refer to someone who has seen and survived much as a "seasoned" person, a veteran. As I watch the 112 students study the 19 cadavers, I am struck by an intersection of generations—grandparents and grandchildren, we might say—in a strange dialogue between the living and the dead, with the instructors in some kind of intermediary parental role. The students' attitudes toward the cadavers evolve over the semester, from fear and anxiety to a form of intimacy through interaction, to, finally, an understanding that the journey together is over. It is time to say good-bye, to send the cadavers to their next stop, while the students move on to holidays, the next semester, the next summer, and whatever lies beyond. During the intense sixteen weeks of the course, the students become seasoned in their approach to the cadaver; it is a time of rapidly maturing emotions, almost forced, as we say of plants that are manipulated to blossom ahead of season.

There is still another sense of the word *season* to speculate upon. If food hasn't gained the desired flavors through preparation, we season it with salt, spices, or herbs, artificially bringing it along to some approximation of "ripeness." Sprinkling the seasoning onto the food quickly changes it. But there is another, more subtle kind of seasoning, the cook's "correcting the seasoning," as he or she samples it and adds seasoning in small amounts until the dish tastes right. I see a parallel in the anatomy lab. First, the students receive the speeded-up version of seasoning as they are thrown into the lab with the immediate task of turning the cadaver over—ready or not. This immersion—through at least the first several dissections—is a rapid sprinkling of experience, like handfuls of fresh ground pepper: the intense view into the body, the consideration of cause of death, the discoveries of scars, disease processes, the wasting of chronic illnesses, and, in general, signs of the many ways the human body can suffer and reach an end to life. In a culture where such topics are often obliquely handled (if not outright ignored), the students confront them suddenly, directly, and vividly. As the semester wears on, the students become much more at home in the lab. They leave the cadaver uncovered more; they work their way through the pelvis and perineum. They talk more freely about the various clues and riddles scattered through the specimens in the lab. They ask about how cadavers got to the lab and where they will go next. By the end of the course—and especially with the final Service of Reflection and Gratitude—the seasoning has been adjusted by further thought and recognition of changes in attitudes throughout the semester. The process will vary from student to student, but I hear many of them recalling the first weeks with a shaking of the head: "I could barely touch the cadaver back then. Boy, we sure have changed!" I hear students acknowledging this development to each other, a crossing of a boundary, a maturation, a seasoning that, as many have said, is a major step toward becoming a physician. I think of the slide of the two men kissing the skeleton; it is an act possible only toward the end of the course.

The kiss suggests the reanimation theme we saw during the middle of the semester: as students abandoned the strictly scientific model for the cadavers, they began to imagine the seasons of life these dead had gone through. Some presentations suggested that the cadavers could still dance, do aerobics, or be part of a poem about Christmas. While this reanimation theme was only a temporary illusion for the cadavers, it parallels the students' more permanent sense of their own revitalization in the death-permeated lab. As in Steve's joke about slipping out of the groove during the bisection of the head, the students reaffirm, successfully and socially, their own sense of life that can, somehow, include and even embrace various forms of death.

The cadavers go on to rejoin the body of the world. In a handful of weeks the hills of Atlanta will change with the arrival of spring. First, crocus and daffodil will sprout and bloom, then japonica and forsythia, then redbud, azaleas, and dogwood. As elegists traditionally point out, the newly dead reenter the procession of the elements and continue the great cycles of nature.

The professors move on to other courses and to their own research projects. In another eight months, they will greet next year's group of freshmen medical students, eager but anxious, some of whom are afraid to touch a cadaver.

The current students are now joyful veterans of Human Anatomy; all 112 who finished the course have successfully passed their exams. Now they head for the holidays, then the spring semester. They move on with a much more complex sense of what the human body contains, a knowledge that is both technical and—as they noticed clues of human experience—wise. Some of the facts they have learned will decay to dormancy or even oblivion, but the deeper truths of the body's intricacies and limitations will stay with them throughout their lifetimes.

And me? My observation in the lab is over. I know that I will never become a physician but that I will spend more of my time writing, especially about medicine and health: it's as if I explored the possibility of one calling and found another, and for this I am thankful. As I have watched the weeks of exploration and clarification, my view of the human body has changed. I feel admiration for the elegant design of the body, its durability, and the subtle variations among each of us human beings. I feel awe for the changes our bodies go through, for the many accidents and ailments that may assail us, and for the final cessation of life, when death overtakes us. If I have been tempted to look at human beings as thinkers only, as mechanical wonders only, as sexual marvels only, now I see better that humanity is more than all of these functions and parts: humanity is rich because of the intertwining of our thoughts and emotions, our spiritual depth, and our physical complexity.

I have followed the journey of my father's remains and I am satisfied that he (and we his family) did the right thing in this donation. I am happy to know — even in approximate fashion — how his body fared at a med school, a place that also cut in the tradition of Vesalius. I have accepted this journey, and more, plumbed it and found it right and good. I am glad to know how he, a professor in life, was a teacher after his death to first-year medical students. A Telemachus in my own fashion, I have been reunited with Odysseus, and we have made our own homecoming. I am able now to celebrate his journey and his fate. For him, there were no provisions for return of ashes to our family, so we could not have a gravestone, nor did we choose to have a memorial marker. Thus the trip to the anatomy lab was for me a quest to pay my respects to his status as cadaver. This book is my memorial to him, something more people will see — and see more deeply — than a weathering gravestone.

His remains were not his living self, of course; I imagine that his soul still exists and perhaps, with the souls of the other donated cadavers, looked down upon the proceedings. Maybe he knows more about the lab than I was able to see. At any rate, I salute whatever existence he has now and feel that some final stages of my mourning and loss have been healed by my adventure in the human anatomy lab. I feel that I know what happened to his body, which is no longer lost to me or to our family; I have traced his path and learned that, if anything, the elements of his body rejoined the natural world more quickly than if he had been buried conventionally. For this, too, I am thankful. I have found a healing in this closure.

And this: when the time for my death comes, I can think of no higher purpose for my muscles and bones, blood vessels and nerves, skin and, yes, even fat, than to send them to a human anatomy lab. I plan for my body to travel to a medical school where a young person, with a scalpel in hand (and perhaps heart in throat) will make a life-changing first cut.

ACKNOWLEDGMENTS

• • •

I'd like to thank several people who helped make this book possible. First is Robert Detweiler, of the Institute of Liberal Arts at Emory University; he directed the Dana Fellows Program that allowed the original research. I would also like to thank the Charles A. Dana Foundation, whose support made my year of study possible. I also thank the twelve other Fellows for that year who provided stimulation and fellowship.

I thank John Stone, M.D., and Arthur W. English, Ph.D., of the Emory University School of Medicine for making possible my observation in the anatomy labs and for their support and friendship. Other instructors in the anatomy program that year who were particularly helpful include Marla B. Luskin, Ph.D.; John K. McDonald, Ph.D.; Lawrence J. Rizzolo, Ph.D.; James R. Wilson, Ph.D.; and Steven L. Wolf, Ph.D. Dr. English and Dr. Wolf read portions of my manuscript; I take responsibility for any errors that remain. I also thank Jerome Sutin, Ph.D., then chair of the Anatomy and Physiology Department.

I also thank Donald G. Shockley, then chaplain of Emory University, and the Rev. Barbara A. B. Patterson, also of Emory, for their contributions.

I would also like to thank Larry R. Churchill, Ph.D., Chair, Social Medicine, School of Medicine, University of North Carolina at Chapel Hill, where I was visiting research professor in 1995–96; while there, I was able to finish work on this book; I thank him and his colleagues, both faculty— including W. D. White, Ph.D., and Barry F. Saunders, M.D.— and staff.

For help and encouragement along the way, I thank Joyce Engelson,

Kathryn M. Lang, Patricia Smith, and Karen Reeds, Drs. Jane Arbuckle Petro and Carolyn Becker, George and Karen Meese, Tom and Marian Price. I thank Profs. Julienne H. Empric and Scott Ward for their colleagueship. I also thank Sally G. Osborne, M.D. I thank members of my family: Nancy, Rebecca, Marjorie, Avise and Luther; Jimmy and Delores, Reid and Dorothy; also, Harvey and Dorothy, Janet and Ian, Marilyn and David, Bette and Sky.

For support from my home institution, Eckerd College, I thank Lloyd W. Chapin, dean of faculty, and Profs. Molly K. Ransbury, Claire A. Stiles, and Thomas E. Bunch, successively chairs of the Creative Arts Collegium, my departmental home. I thank work-scholars for their faithful help: Maite B. Diez, Kari Jarde Hoblitzell, Alison Creighton, and Heather Furrow.

I thank especially my excellent agent, Ann Rittenberg, for bringing this book to publication and my gifted editor at Picador, George Witte; both offered fine suggestions to improve the book.

I thank all of the first-year class over whose shoulders I looked at the School of Medicine, Emory University. I especially thank the six students at table Number 3, David Carlton, Lisa Cerilli, Steven Grant, Cliff Grossman, Jonathan Kalish, and Jocelyne Oriole. I have used five pseudonyms (Miss Y, Lex, Fred, Todd, and Sam) to protect the privacy of actual persons. Mrs. X, in Dr. English's lecture, is a made-up character. All quotations attributed to persons have been checked with them for accuracy and propriety.

I thank Dover Publications, Inc., for permission to reproduce the Vesalius engravings, Arthur W. English for the two drawings from the *Human Anatomy Course Syllabus,* and Karl Jacobs for his linocut of the human heart.

I thank the persons who donated their bodies and their families for their contributions to medical education and research. These wonderful gifts are the heart of the human anatomy lab.

—A. H. C.